A **CRAZY PROFESSOR** TELLS ALMOST
ALL THE **ADVENTURES** AND **MISADVENTURES** OF
HIS LIFE IN **PSYCHOLOGY**

PSYCHOLOGY CONFIDENTIAL

JOHN E. MARTIN, PH.D.

Copyright © 2021 by John E. Martin.

All rights reserved. This book or any portion thereof may not be reproduced or used in any manner whatsoever without the express written permission of the publisher except for the use of brief quotations in a book review.

All Dog/Cat pair pictures provided by Animal Wellness Center of OC, Costa Mesa, CA (animalwellnessoc.com)

All professor pictures, and professional photography refining of other pictures throughout, provided by JohnWatkinsphotographer.com

Publishing Services provided by Paper Raven Books
Printed in the United States of America
First Printing, 2021

Paperback ISBN= 978-1-7376131-0-7
Hardback ISBN= 978-1-7376131-1-4

REVIEWS

What Others Have Said (or Should Have) about This Outstanding Book and Author

"He can compress the most words into the smallest idea of any man I [n]ever met."

—Abraham Lincoln

"In every fat book there is a thin book trying to get out [like yours]."

—Unknown and none of your business

"Sometimes when reading [it] I have a paralyzing suspicion that he is trying to be funny."

—Guy Davenport

"Your life story would not make a good book. Don't even try [oops, too late]."

—Fran Liebowitz

"The beautiful part of writing is that you don't have to get it right the first time [like this one]…unlike, say, a brain surgeon."

—Robert Cormier

"The covers of this book are too far apart."

—Ambrose Bierce

> "There are two kinds of books: those that no one reads and those that no one ought to read [such as this one]."
>
> —H. L. Mencken

> "If I were given the opportunity to present a gift to the next generation, it would be the ability for each individual to learn to laugh at himself [and at this laughable book]."
>
> —Charles M. Schulz

> "If you have to pay the bills, and you write something you're not proud of [like this], use a pen name for that [oops again]."
>
> —Dean Koontz

> "There's no thief like a bad book."
>
> —Italian Proverb

DEDICATION

I dedicate this book to the four most wonderful and beautiful women who have been in my life—Vera Martin (my mother), Rebecca Martin, Lucia Cheng, and Catherine Liu Martin—who at important stages in it, cared for, blessed, encouraged, put up with, and loved me, nonetheless.

I thank you from the reaches of my new heart.
With Great Love,
John

A WACKY PSYCHOLOGY PROFESSOR'S INSIDE STORY

*True Confessions, Mad Professions,
Mishaps, and Hilarity,
Along His and Psychology's
Strange, Crooked Path to
Wisdom and Sanity,
Healing, Faith, and Fun*

TABLE OF CONTENTS

I. **Parking Garage (Level P1)—Welcome to the Book**   1
   a. Parking P1a (Blue Zone). *About the Book*   1
   b. Parking P1b (Red Zone). *Special Note to the (Potential) Reader*   3

II. **First Floor—Welcome to Psychology**   5
   a. Room 101. *Psychology: What's Up?*   7
   b. Room 102. *The Tour*   15

III. **Second Floor—Welcome to the University**   19
   a. Room 201. *Finding Psychology*   21
   b. Room 202. *Early Psych Grad Student Life*   29
   c. Room 203. *Welcome to the Doctoral Program*   49
   d. Room 204. *Psychology Teaching Trials*   65

IV. **Third Floor—Psychological Adventures and Misadventures**   87
   a. Room 301. *Clinical Consultation Psychology*   89
   b. Room 302. *Training Travails and Research Fun*   107
   c. Room 303. *World-Traveling Professor*   125

V. **Fourth Floor—Psychology of Life and Family Living**   143
   a. Room 401. *Animal Psychology*   145
   b. Room 402. *Child and Family Psychology*   173

VI. **Fifth Floor—Psychology of Trauma**   213
   a. Room 501. *Veterans, Trauma, and PTSD*   215
   b. Room 502. *Personal Trauma Confessions*   231
   c. Room 503. *Trauma Coping, Therapy, and Recovery*   251

VII. **Sixth Floor—Professions—Beyond Psychology**   261
   a. Room 601. *The Psychology of Hope and Faith*   263
   b. Room 602. *Spiritual Integration Crossroads*   275

VIII. Seventh Floor—Psychological Reflections   309
    a.   Room 701. *So What Now?*   311
    b.   Room 702. *Exit Right—Some Final Parting Thoughts*   317

Bonus Room 800: Psychological Postscript   319
    Author Postscript: *From Academic to Writer*   319

More About Dr. John   327

Acknowledgements   329

References   331

WELCOME TO THE BOOK

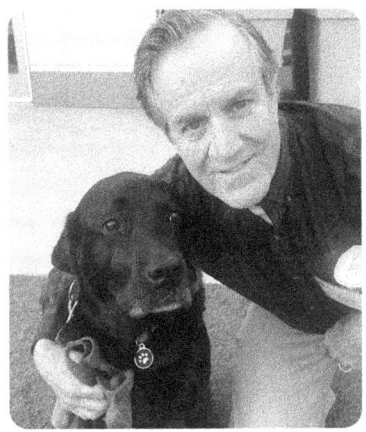

"Life can only be understood backward; but it must be lived forwards"
— SOREN KIERKEGAARD

About the Book

This book is all about my life as a very peculiar sort of clinical psychologist and professor, finding, living in, sailing, and sinking on the waters of an outrageous career across hospitals, clinics, universities, research programs, world travels, and crazy animal and family tales.

In it, I'll take you to all those places, people, and times—and *man* (am I allowed to use this gender-specific term?) do I have stories to tell!

SPECIAL NOTE TO THE (POTENTIAL) READER
(that's you, right?)

You should know that this book you are about to read and experience has been constructed and impersonated as a semi-directed tour through the world of psychology—led by me, your author, the crazy professor tour guide. By the way, I can't think of anyone better to give it, can you? Don't answer that. For our tour, should you choose to take it, I have creatively chosen to employ a lame metaphor—a building (you know it's not actually there) that I brilliantly call "Psychology." In it are seven different floors, illustrated here in chapter form (since this is a book after all), stacked one upon another (that's how a building, though probably not psychology, works), representing seven areas of psychology (and anti-psychology, I might add) that I know a bit about, have lived in and around, and more or less survived.

The seven floors are subdivided into rooms covering various areas in the field, its study, practice, and my peculiar experience in psychology. Each room you will tour has at least something to do with that floor's overall theme. So as not to bore you entirely, like many of the courses you have taken in school, I tell the story of psychology principally according to my own wild and crazy *insider's* view—confidentially, of course. I've used lots of embellishing stories, illustrations, true confessions, and professions to which you might relate (many of you will, I'm guessing). Hopefully, you will at least appreciate them, if not find them interesting, or, you never know, highly enjoyable. This is not to mention "educational." Okay, maybe not the latter.

Dare to find out? Yes?

...Then let's get started!

FIRST FLOOR

WELCOME TO PSYCHOLOGY

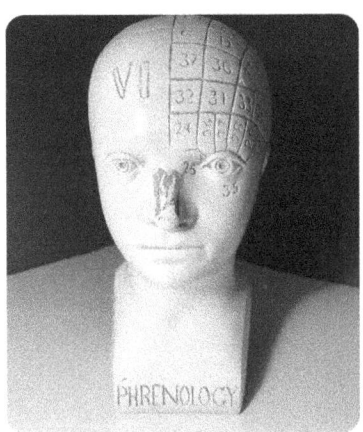

<u>Psy-chol-o-gy</u>
*"The science that tells you what you already know,
using words that you can't understand."*

—UNKNOWN

We start out on this first floor as a pre-tour step (if you haven't read the special note to the reader a couple pages back, you will have no idea what this "floor" business is about. Now go back and read it). Here, we will find out if and why you might be interested in psychology (and reading this book, no less) before you get dragged into reading it (my goal). To that end, I wanted to be thorough, probably too thorough as you will discover, going over the various reasons and motivations of why one like you would want anything to do with psychology. Indeed, there are many good reasons. You might learn something—perhaps even why you want, or should want, something to do with psychology. That information alone would be worth the trouble, don't you think? I do. You especially might find a strange, curious, perhaps crazed interest in psychology that I've not been able to talk you out of. Want to see? Let's proceed together then to Room 101, appropriately numbered as our introduction to psychology.

ROOM 101

PSYCHOLOGY: WHAT'S UP?

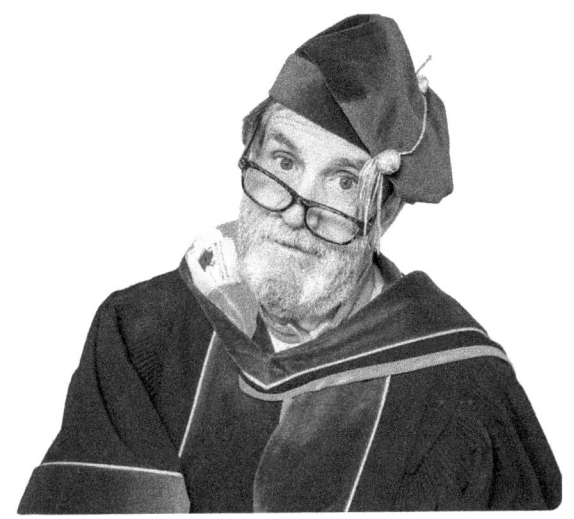

All professor pictures provided by johnwatkinsphotographer.com

Sometimes I lie awake at night and ask, 'Where have I gone wrong?' Then a voice says to me, 'This is going to take more than one night.'"

—Charles M. Schulz

What's up with you and psychology? "Good question!" was my favorite reply to those thousands of student questioners over so many years of teaching. You know and have heard the phrase, "There are good ones, not so good ones," and, of course, stupid ones (the questions, not the students—though to be honest they both could be). As the proverbial "they" say, there are no dumb questions, only dumb answers. Here's a secret: What do we professorial types say when we have *no* idea what or how to answer?— "Good question!"

These admissions notwithstanding, I do hope to spare you further indignity with my answers here, as your (proverbial again) Psychology Answer Man and would-be Guide into the World of Psychology—Le Tour we are about to embark upon. That is, should you accept this invitation to see the field and practice of psychology like never before, through my eyes and strange mind.

BUT, what's that they say?—you can't unsee those things you wish you had never seen. So, beware. The way you will view psychology after reading this book, and taking my strange and crazy tour through it, will be forever changed, carrying with it the risk of possibly ruining psychology to you and yours from now on such that you will want nothing to do with psychology ever again! Consider yourself sternly warned.

So, let's start at the beginning—before our tour commences—to see if I can give you a few persuasive, though possibly stupid, answers to those broad questions: What about psychology, and why should you be interested in reading a book about it by an "insider" like me, pursuing a career in it, or deciding whether or not to use psychology in some way in your life? That is, if you haven't already, fortunately or unfortunately, done it.

The answers are all there within the big looming building standing before us, in our way, actually—like when your spouse, girlfriend, boyfriend, fiancé, or parent drags you in for psychological counseling over some issue that is *all their fault*. You will notice the giant Greek Ψ (this stands for "psychology") emblazoned as a warning of sorts on the building façade. There, you will be guided, floor-by-floor and room-by-room, to areas, departments, divisions, and crazy stories about the field and practice of psychology that you may or may not know much about. I'm assuming the latter, but you must forgive me should you be the former. I can work with both of you.

You will hear and learn about the strange people and animals of psychology, including your incorrigible insider tour guide, and some interesting revelations on the "tricks of the trade," bizarre history, and zany maneuvers of the field. I promise it will be worth it. If it's not, then fire me just like I encourage my clients to do so after even a single session of therapy (some did). Similarly, this may be a time for you to ask for a book refund (it's still not too late).

> **READER ALERT #1:** You will be seeing these warning label alarm messages throughout the book, so PAY ATTENTION—at least more than we did to the warnings on the cigarette packs in the 1960s.
>
> *Maybe you have read just far enough to decide this is not the book for you. Though I think it is, only you can decide. If you've decided it's not, then this is probably the place to consider demanding a full refund.*

You're still here?

How about if I try to convince you to follow me through some of my possibly brilliant, educational (maybe not) reasoning, professorial expertise, and captivating stories with delightful entertainment along the way? That's my goal.

But wait…before entering the psych building, can we talk about those three big pending questions demanding our answer: Why psychology? Why you? and Why me? Or, in this case, why *this* book about psychology and *your analysis.* I'm sure you've wondered, and maybe were too afraid to investigate on your own or inquire of a professional like me. There's nothing to be fearful of, excepting what we might find out about you. Nevertheless, why don't we give it a try.

Everything You Wanted to Know about Psychology but Were Afraid to Ask

As a psychologist who is trained in evaluating people probabilities, not to mention "psychoanalyzing" your particularly strange behavior and appearance, I'm imagining you have most likely experienced psychology in any of the following ways:

First (Reason #1), you were a consumer who bought or used pop, self-help psychology books or programs for self-improvement (no need to feel guilty, we all have succumbed to this).

Second (Reason #2), you have performed frenetic internet searches on psychological issues, topics, and problems you've wondered or desperately needed to know about (no judgment here either, since of course you have).

Third (Reason #3), you've sought out and attended talks, seminars, or workshops/retreats for things like how to be motivated and change your darn self and others too. Now please don't tell me you've fallen for that rapid, no-sweat hypnotism "cure," or worse yet from a stage hypnotist like I once feared I did!

Fourth (Reason #4), you've suffered (okay, maybe "suffer" is not the best word choice here) through therapy for relationship problems, addiction treatment, or other life and personal issues in need of fixing.

If you are like me, you've "accomplished" all four, so no judgment here. Good for us. But I'm not done. There's one, and maybe two or three more to consider, if you will. We will.

Fifth (Reason #5) reason of interest (my definition of ROI), some, though certainly not you, would argue that their personal, psychological ROI evolved from the scientific deduction that their many problems were someone else's fault. For example, your parents (duh), your parents' parents (to the "fourth generation," according to no less than the Bible!), the government (no doubt), your spouse (kiss-kiss), or heaven forbid, your wounded and bratty "inner child" who refuses to grow up and get over it!

But my more lighthearted fun here is not to discount or minimize the real tragedies of our lives that so many of us have experienced and lived through—being deeply hurt, damaged, wounded, or abused by others *and* our own self, resulting in true emotional and psychological trauma, bitterness, and lasting harm to ourselves and those close to us. These personal and relationship devastators occupy an all-too-large portion of psychology's world for us, and this book does not shy away from such revelations and confessions.

Sixth (Bonus ROI Reason #6). I'm not done yet? Nope. There's this last Big One I can't neglect. I promise no more after this. This sixth, most common but no doubt foolish, cause of psychological "interest"—or entrapment, we might say—is in some ways the most insidious: TAKING A PSYCHOLOGY CLASS. You may have semiconsciously, or fully consciously but foolhardily, accepted the *dance* invitation to the psychology ball—like so many students of mine who have taken a college or university psychology course from me.

Here are some relatively weak but still persuasive explanations for your Number Six ROI, psychology class entrapment:

You most likely:

a. had to take a psychology course—Intro Psych 101, for example—to fulfill a degree requirement for your subject major;

b. decided for some nonsensical reason to major in psychology and had to take many psych courses all the way from near useless to those that are not so much fun, like experimental statistics (arrrgh);

c. thought a psych course would be a more interesting and easier "A" or "B" grade-point booster (wrong on both counts);

d. saw it was the only course still available (a very bad sign, if you know what I mean), and you had to take one for your full load necessary to stay in school and for your scholarship requirement, or;

e. decided to just enroll in one because some well-intended (now ex-) friend or (horrors) a professor told you so.

Speaking of professors, may I introduce a seventh, extra special add-on reason? Thanks, I will. I know I promised "no more," but I lied. Just this one. Now this last reason for one's interest in psychology is not for you more normal people. It's for those folks like your author who are more *responsible* for causing disappointment and psychological harm to you and likely the field of psychology too—other professors of psychology and psychiatry. Come to think of it, why would my colleagues and maybe professorial friends from the university and medical school want to read or have *anything* to do with this book? Another "good question."

Well, just to take a wild stab at it, there is the fellow psychologist's, psychiatrist's, or therapist's prurient interest in catching all those things I'm lying to you about. There are some, but not enough to be worried over or that I haven't warned you about. For example, you were there or recognize yourself from the actual stories I've distorted, exaggerated, or made up. But the opposite might be the case—you just want to enjoy an outrageous, hilarious rendition of your crazy career and life in psychology or psychiatry. If the latter, good. Read on.

Final Answer

I am now ready to answer that profound question: What about psychology, and, relatedly, why this book (and tour guide, me)? *Are you a fit? Do you qualify? Are you still interested in reading?* **You qualify. You are hereby approved for the tour.** This was what's known as a "surprise quiz." Rest assured—nobody fails.

Incidentally, if you checked "yes" to even one of the six psychological reasons and qualifications for interest in psychology and this tour (I'm purposely ignoring you ROI #7s. I'm only speaking from now on to the normal people), that would have been sufficient for entrance to the psychology building we are approaching.

You might be surprised (well, maybe not) to know that I, too, ran after or stumbled into all seven of the psychology interest cake-baited bear traps—but not the stage hypnotist part, which I refuse to admit. Traps were flung open, having done their job, so to speak, and I wandered into and through many psychological adventures and misadventures. But I'm not quite done with my psychoanalysis of you and me. May I continue?

So, admit it: psychology has impacted your life and/or the life of your family and friends, ultimately in some major ways, and hopefully more for good than bad. And, let's be honest, you want to find out what is so darn wrong with you—and especially those other crazy family members, friends, and coworkers—but were afraid to ask! Right? That would be my first guess about you, the professional client-reader.

But on the other hand, maybe you are just interested in peeking behind that curtain cloaking the strange and mysterious field of psychology. You're curious and want to know what's up with all the talk and obsession over psychology—and we are indeed a society obsessed with psych-e-ology, as a pastor friend of mine once sarcastically called it. You would be my second reader guess, the psychological voyeur.

I confess, my favorite target audience, readership-wise, consists of those of you looking for laughable or ridiculous stories about psychology, as retold by your wacky professor author (look again at the cover picture if you don't believe me). Be honest, that is why you got the book. I am your humorous insider who will tickle and occasionally shock you with a bunch of Dave Barry–esque stories and wacky confessions from my student, teaching, "professoring," and world travel days, as well as my strange family and goofy animals. That would make you reader target three, the entertainment seeker.

And finally, my fourth guess would include those of you who are more serious about exploring those deeper places, revelations, and confessions from the all-too-human person beneath the professor's doctoral robe and behind his pontificating pulpit and therapist couch. You are hoping, and will not be disappointed, for an invite into my personal struggles, traumas, breakdowns, and breakthroughs along the way as I share my strange, crooked path to healing and wisdom at times, in spite of psychology. This book should give you a private look behind the curtain, revealing a variety of unvarnished truths about the inner and outer workings of your author and his field—the good, the not-so-good, and the occasionally nonsensical. You, then, are my personal story investigator-reader.

Through it all—the tour, stories, conversational asides, lame humor, and entertainment attempts—I plan to serve as your teacher (hopefully), mentor (that's going too far, sir), therapist (possibly), research lecturer (sleeping not allowed), and world travel guide (fasten your seatbelts and place your seat back tray into its original upright position). It should be an educational ride, and, if not, at least mildly entertaining.

ROOM 102

THE TOUR

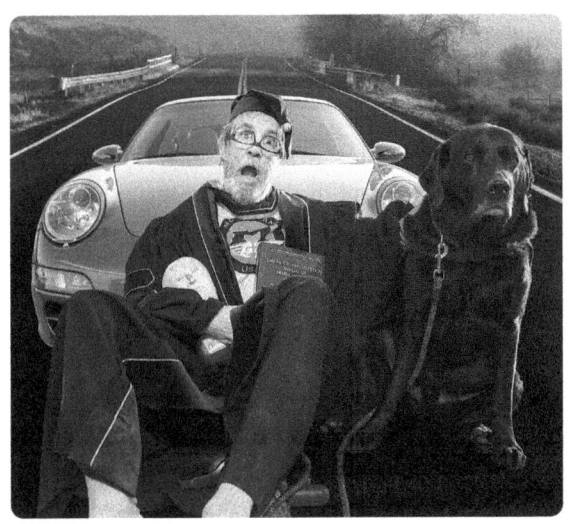

"You should always leave the party [or tour] 10 minutes before you actually do."

—GARY LARSON

Whichever psychology-seeker, participant, and book-reader categories you fall into, you've read this far and are hereby agreeing to some basic informed consent, HIPAA compliant, risk awareness, and harm liability release (to me, that is). You have, haven't you? May I assume, then, you are ready to take the tour of my psychological and professorial revelations and meanderings shared (confidentially) from behind the student's desk, the professor's podium, the therapist's couch, and the researcher's laboratory and world travels? Good. So, get ready for quite a ride.

Psychology Tour Map

All right. Now you are about to enter the world of psychological adventures and misadventures, teaching travails, strange travels, crazy family, and goofy animal psychology stories. As your tour guide, I'll be leading you into and through the portal of Ψ, as outlined in the Table of Contents, which you may or may not have even looked at. No matter. Nobody fails this course.

Anyway, let's make our way to that grand building you see before you—with that Greek Ψ plaque above the front entrance—and its seven main floors representing key areas of psychology. Kind of like Noah's ark, the psychology building is also sufficiently large to contain all the psychological arenas, stories, experiences, and imaginations of your author-professor-guide—at least the parts he's most interested in, had something to do with, and has translated into chapters for you.

> **TOUR/READER ALERT #2:** You can set your own pace and take your OWN TOUR! You don't need me. *You* get to decide which floors and areas are of most interest to you, which are not, and can start there with *no penalty*. The Table of Contents with its page numbers can assist you in this. You can catch up with us on another floor later if you'd like (we won't be going so quickly that you can't find us). Or not.

Since you are the reader, and it is still a free country (last I checked), go ahead and jump to the sections and chapters you find most interesting, curious, crazy, or strange, and begin with those, until you get bored or irritated (or both) enough to jump to another one of interest—or quit reading entirely. The book and stories do not require having been to a previous floor or topic area, though you would find the book and tour have been laid out in sections, paths, and chapters that follow a general chronology, time frame, and logic.

If you do decide to jump around, have fun, but good luck with that. Otherwise, I suggest you hang with me as we go through the general floor-by-floor and area-by-area journey that has been laid out properly. Then, at the end, if dissatisfied, bored, irritated, outraged, and/or (re)traumatized, you may set the book (not me) on fire (I'll even help!) and mail the ashes to me for appropriate application as fertilizer for my garden.

One last warning: You might have deduced that these various floors represent most of the areas and points of interest on the magnificent psychological map. But as your grand tour guide, I get to regurgitate my own, many psychological and academic pontifications, confessions, justifications, illuminations, imaginations, and entertainments I once foisted on my students, colleagues, friends, and family members. Now I get to foist them (I like this word) on you! Yippee!

Mini Tour Appetizer
As your itinerant teacher for this journey into and through the (actually, *my*) world of psychology, we will be starting with my crazy psychology student and graduate years, including my sentence (only partly commuted) as a child and hospital psychologist. This was followed by time as a tottering (no, not doddering, but that could work) wet-behind-the-ears VA staff psychologist, the (unable to escape) bizarre imprisonment in the college and university teaching circus and goofy professor world, and as an administratively challenged department administrator, which fortunately I've mainly blotted from my consciousness and this book. Then comes the meandering trail and trials of a would-be clinical and community researcher here and abroad. Last, and maybe least, I'll subject you to stories from my firepit barefooted run as a committed (or I should be) Christian psychologist, pastor, and mission worker to Africa, Romania, Mexico, South Korea, and North Korea (all right, I'm lying about the North part, though that would have been a story—a book written from a North Korean jail cell!).

Getting back to you. Since you presumably bought the book or stole it (hopefully not), you ought to get a money's-worth tour for laying down that hard-earned cash. As infamously said by Joan Rivers, "Can we talk?" I plan to use that device to talk more directly to you in some private asides throughout the tour. I will be giving you those special, priceless secrets, wisdoms, and not-such-wisdoms you would never hear from any other psychologist or professor.

> **CAN WE TALK?**
> This is the dialogue box I warned you about, and you will be seeing throughout the book—a place where I can take you aside and confide in you some particular wisdoms, or nonsense, about what it all means, what to make of it or watch out for, what's funny, what's not, and how I think you could use or misuse some stuff from that chapter or section. So look out for these hopefully entertaining, if not educating, private confidences.

Let the Tour Commence

If you will follow me to the elevators—I think I can fit you all in—I will lead you to and through the seven floors of psychology that touch or have importantly affected your lives, and mine of course.

Leaving the first floor, our Welcome to Psychology that we have been meandering around for a while, we're about to be regurgitated onto the second floor—Welcome to the University. There, I'll be admitting how I first fell or was sucked into it all. Perhaps you might relate to or appreciate the crooked path there, but even if not, I think you might like my outlandish experiences finding and *becoming psychology* (so to speak) quite some time ago (I'm not telling how long ago, but you industrious snoops can figure that out).

SECOND FLOOR

WELCOME TO THE UNIVERSITY

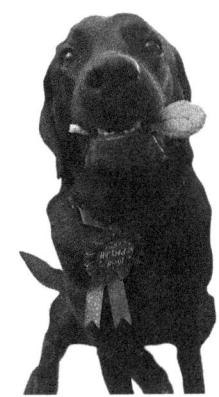

*"Education is what survives
when what has been learned has been forgotten."*

—B.F. Skinner

Most all of us have had experiences during, related to, or *caused* by university or college life on our own, or vicariously through our family, friends, or coworkers. "It's all good" is a phrase I've heard some use, but it was not "all good" for me in my journey to and through the world of psychology. Maybe you will relate to the story of finding the psychology of the university or graduate school. My college days were mostly a blur, since I didn't take any psychology courses as an undergraduate, so I don't have much to say about that, except for some trauma I will discuss later. On the other hand, I do have plenty of fun stories about my *teaching* psychology to my college and university undergraduates, so stay tuned. Let's jump into the story of how one should *not* try to "find" psychology the way I did.

ROOM 201

FINDING PSYCHOLOGY

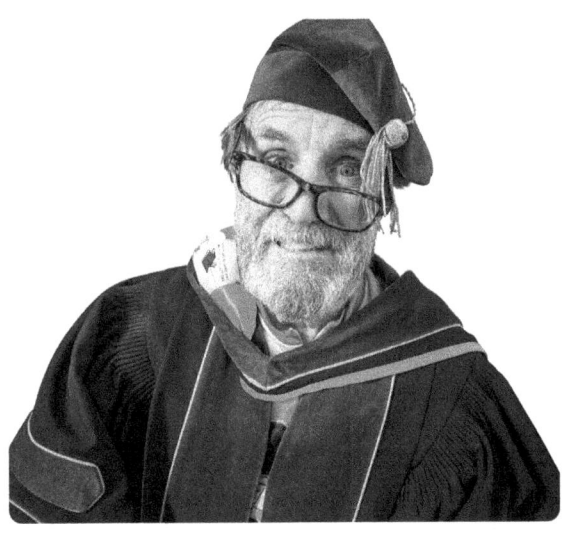

"If opportunity doesn't knock, build a door."
—Milton Berle

I was most unceremoniously "welcomed" to psychology through a strange and, you might say, providential door when I finally decided to check in to this "Hotel Psychology" (thank you, Eagles). As the song goes, I somehow could never seem to check out and leave despite multiple attempts. Like addiction. To be honest, my traumatic experiences in childhood, those with my father, and those in college led me to my interest in psychology. Maybe like you (okay, maybe not), I needed to find out what was so ridiculously wrong with me, and I thought perhaps psychology could tell me, if not fix me. Instead, it sucked me into a different kind of psychological quicksand and a world that had no apparent exit and no doorway or floor-lit sign to guide me. It was all in or all out, as I discovered.

Welcome—Not! (Don't Call Us, We'll Call You)

It was the fall of 1969, and recently graduated from college, I was politely but firmly directed to the psychology department's office door. "Don't let the door hit you on the way out" might (or should) have been said.

I had just ventured over from the graduate school of education, where I spent my first and only day in class in their master's in educational psychology—mainly teachers vying for their degree in guidance and counseling. At best, the fellow grad students were there to follow a noble calling to help students with their counseling needs, but possibly just to get a higher salary with their master's degree and get back at all those students who had made their lives so miserable in the classroom. Okay, I retract that last part (but it might be true). Anyway, I knew that department wasn't for me. I had no interest in working in the schools, counselor or not, especially after my experience in college taking the teachers' education block and watching my favorite teacher and mentor get treated so terribly by their school administrators.

On the other hand, I'd heard and read a lot about psychology, not to mention my brief and relatively unsuccessful experience of therapy in college. I was curious and thought psychology might be a better fit, and perhaps a refuge of sorts, from the pull and pursuit of my father's radio business and his strong-willed efforts to entrap me in it all. I did major in business and economics, so I decided to at least give the radio craft and my father's new business a try—to his great pleasure—that is, until my radio days came to an embarrassing ambush.

It was a classic double approach–avoidance conflict—as we say in the field. I wanted to please my father, and was afraid not to, *and* I didn't want to please him. Then, I was drawn, totally unprepared, toward psychology for both my healing and collateral distancing from Dad, while at the same time being frightened of it for what it might show me about myself. Confused? So was I. And I certainly couldn't imagine starting a *career* in psychology!

Have you ever had the kind of conflict where you were torn, sucked, and repelled at the same time about directions in your life? Come on, admit it, you have. By the way, psychology has lots to say about that sort of thing, and many of our clients come in that state too—highly ambivalent, stuck or unable to decide, and often depressed and anxious about it. That was me. Nevertheless, I decided to give radio the ole college try.

Radio Daze
Here's how it went for me, how I broke out of my ambivalence, funny stories and all. My halfhearted attempts to resolve the life-and-dad (no, not "death," though some days it felt that way) conflict, please my father, and become that dutiful son in his footsteps began with summers during my college years. I was ambivalent at the least, but still looking for ways to kind of please my father, but ultimately displease him by finding my own way in life without his harsh hand.

So I agreed to be rotated around the various jobs, roles, and departments across the radio stations Dad had purchased and moved across the country to run. These included man-on-the-street interviewer for a show called "Speak Out," a newscaster/reader over the air, traffic secretary (no, not out on the street, silly, but the one who typed out all the radio program schedules for the week), commercial producer, and (my favorite) DJ. My radio "personality" for my late-night acid rock program was "Dr. John's Nite Trip" (named after my Louisiana Cajun hero, Dr. John the Nite Tripper). Funny, the name I drew out of my tinfoil radio beam hat was strangely prophetic—I'm now known to a number of my friends, and some clients, as "Dr. John"—a relatively kind, familiar, and even humorous but accurate personal moniker.

This was my junior year's summer with my father at the radio station, and I decided to carry it further by volunteering at the college radio station, and then at the city one. I volunteered as a newsperson and DJ at the college station, combined with my time as a very bad radio ad salesman for the city station. While I never made a single sale, I was "promoted" to be an all-night radio babysitter and DJ when their weekend person either quit or was fired. I never did find out.

My job was mostly "babysitting" the broadcasts, in which I monitored and controlled the taped shows, read the news, and helped the early Sunday morning preachers air their sermons. Sometimes it was fun. I recall one preacher—a real hellfire and brimstone screamer—who didn't have such a good sense of microphone etiquette. He was in an adjoining glass-enclosed booth, where I could watch and cue him, and he loved to alternate his voice and distance to and from the microphone throughout the half-hour show. If I didn't know better, I'd have thought he was having fun with *me*.

At one point, he would be whispering to the listening audience (however few there were) from far away from the microphone, and *then*, in a flash, run to the microphone and scream into it some critical scripture or call to Christian action! Riding the "pot" or the volume control was a real treat with this guy. If I hadn't taken my job so seriously, I would have recognized the great humor in it. (One sleepy early morning, I forgot to turn the volume on, and there was "dead air" for about 15 minutes until I woke up, noticed my error, and suddenly turned it up with ear-piercing shock and mid-sentence nonsense for the listener! I didn't get any calls, so maybe his listening audience was pretty close to or actually zero. No worries. I never confessed this to him. But God knew.)

Then there was the *pièce de résistance* that made the choice between a career in radio and *anything* else. I had just left a Saturday night party at my fraternity, feeling pretty good, I might add, arriving before midnight for my 12 to 7 AM show. It wasn't long after that I received the call.

I was getting settled behind the radio operations panel, a large broadcasting microphone in front of me, big reel-to-reel tape recorders to either side for prerecorded shows to babysit, and glass-enclosed booths for individual speakers and radio shows. I controlled the buttons, including whether the mics were live as well as the volume.

The call came in, and it was "Sergeant Smith" from the police city desk. He urgently needed me to put out an emergency bulletin over the airways. He said there was a RACE RIOT going on in the southeast part of the city, and they were asking all residents to keep away from their windows and lock their doors. Shocked, I said I couldn't do that—it would create a panic! But he insisted and said it was now a police order. So, of course, I complied. Within a few minutes, I had written out the bulletin that I read over the airways, punctuated with the beep, beep, beep special bulletin sounds in the background and scary warning, attention-getting audio. I was required to keep in the things about door locks and staying away from windows, and the police "sergeant" wouldn't let me change "race riot" to "major disturbance," as I fearfully suggested. So I left it in, unfortunately.

After the "race riot" bulletin aired, the phone lines lit up, furiously! I began to answer them and got an earful of terrorized questions. Sanity briefly flew by my consciousness, and I decided to call the police back. They knew of *no* Sergeant Smith or any kind of a disturbance anywhere in their smaller midwestern farming city. "Uh-oh. S---."

As I began crafting my cancellation of the previous race riot bulletin—trying vainly to construct something that wouldn't make me sound like the *complete idiot I was*—another call came in that I decided to take for some reason. It was "Junior" and there was uproarious laughter in the background. It was the fraternity party I had left an hour ago, still going strong, now in renewed hilarity! Junior tried to apologize for the "joke" turned serious by my idiocy and tried at a serious but phony "concern" for my terrible predicament. All I could say was—brilliantly I might add—"I hate you, Junior, and never want to talk to you ever again!" I wanted to kill him. In a way, I still do, setting aside the positive effect it had on my finding a career in psychology and not radio. Okay, I'm kidding about killing him. I might just thank him if he is reading this, but he owes me a beer.

So, I returned to my re-bulletin, finished it, and enacted the "special bulletin" beeping alert from radio station XXX. And I read it. It went something like, "We have cancelled the previous bulletin about the city disturbance due to the fact that it could not be confirmed by the police. You are in no danger, so you may go by your windows and unlock your doors." Stupid.

When I told my radio station magnate father on the phone about this days later, he, after laughing for a good while, asked me, "Why didn't you call the police to verify the call? That is standard procedure in something like this." *Now* you tell me!

But this embarrassing lesson was not over. A standard procedure when something like this happens over the airways (an FCC regulation of some sort) is to write a detailed problem, incident, or "irregularity" report. So I did and left it on the desk of the program director that night, hoping when they fired me it would be in private. But for a couple weeks, I heard nothing. Maybe the report got lost in the shuffle of paperwork or dropped accidentally into the round file. I was free, sigh of relief! But not so.

When I came in during the day at the end of two weeks to pick up my (probably last) paycheck, there was a gaggle of salesmen down at the end of the main office, snickering as I passed by them. Then I heard: "Hey John, had any race riots lately?" Uproarious laughter! They loved it! (Reminded me of the crazy comedy sitcom, *WKRP in Cincinnati*.) I was humiliated, and my budding radio career was over. Though I was not fired, I fired myself from any future career or anything to do with radio (or Dad, of course).

Next Floor: Psychology!

I was fearful as I slunk into the department's main office and sat down, waiting to be noticed. The head secretary (probably the department chair's tough senior secretary) raised her head and asked how she could help me (not really wanting to, I perceived, but there was no one else to get rid of me, so she was "it"). I explained my situation and my interest in becoming a graduate student there, using way too many words (as one does when they are fearful and know they are about to be rejected). But she stopped me mid-sentence and said I would need to talk to someone in the admissions committee, or their administrative secretary. I got the latter.

Our "interview" was efficiently quick—too quick as it turned out. It didn't take this trying-to-be-nice (not really) but stern admissions "guardian" much time to recognize that this would not take long at all. Here's the crazy (or stupid) part that I expressed with great sincerity and hopeful "qualification": I had never taken even a single undergraduate course in psychology, but I had done a lot of reading about psychology and was "highly motivated for having a possible career in it" (thinking, no doubt, that would be persuasive). That should be enough, right?

To make matters even more ridiculous, I asked this incredulous, possibly shocked listener for a paid assistantship as well. I had no job and needed the money. Outrageous, no? Pay this completely unprepared and unimpressive student and accept him into your more rigorous program in experimental psych? Yeah, right.

Getting what was coming to me, I received that not so much "soft no," but more like a "get out of here, and stop wasting our time with this foolish application!" Given my outstanding qualifications, the answer should have been to throw me out of the building, or at minimum a stinging rebuke of: "Get out of here, you fool! How stupid do you think we are?"

My slinky stooped shoulder entrance became my exit. I wasn't really that surprised, but I felt sad and defeated. "Now what…" was my following week's depressed musings. But while I was what you could call "psyched out" and kicked out of psychology forever, something crazy happened.

Providence or Coincidence?
A week after I was so unceremoniously ushered to the psychology department exit, I received a life-redirecting (and redefining) call: "Would you be available to come in and talk with us about entering our program? We've had one of our graduate assistants not return (ends up she was in Hawaii and decided not to come back—lucky woman!) and we need someone *right away*." They didn't say, or have to say, you were our *only* candidate. So foolishly, I came in.

My other alternative in life, as I've mentioned, was to work for and under my dad in his radio stations following my college graduation. He wanted me to learn all about the business and hopefully one day take over. But my radio daze experiences took care of that conflict. I was a mess emotionally and psychologically, and my relationship with my father was far from good, as you will learn.

So, psychology drew me, both accidentally and purposefully, together. First, I wanted to find out what was so wrong with me. Second, I had done much reading in it and wanted to learn more. Third, I hoped to retain my student deferment from the draft (this was Vietnam War time). Lastly, I thought it could be that refuge from Dad's pressure to join the business.

My radio days daze now past, I enrolled in the master's program in psychology. I continued to live in the town where the two radio stations and my father's company were and stayed at home until my psychologist and major professor at school threatened to no longer see me in counseling if I didn't move out. I was pretty messed up with anxiety and unresolved issues with Dad, so I did. It was a reprieve and ultimately a blessing.

ROOM 202

EARLY PSYCH GRAD STUDENT LIFE

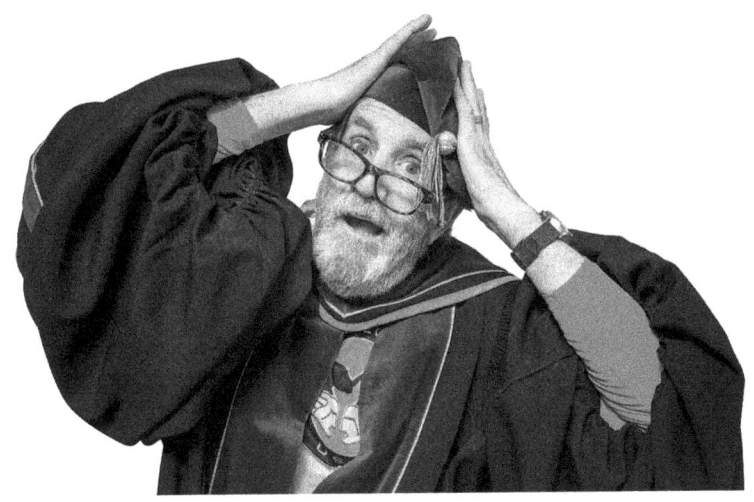

"When you come to a fork in the road, take it."
—Yogi Berra

What in the world to do? Think now, John. After dodging the "bullet" of a likely irredeemable career in radio broadcasting (thank God for crazy radio daze), and advertising terrible products nobody wants or needs while working for and under my fear-inducing father, I hustled back into the protective custody of school—graduate school in psychology. At least there was that.

Welcome to Graduate School—The Student Years I

Upon entrance to the master's program in experimental psychology, it didn't take long for me to be rudely awakened to the differences between the life of the liberal arts college student and a graduate student in a science-based experimental psychology program. Though it was only a master's program, it was still a big step for me, especially given my mushy science-allergic brain.

Anxiously, I appeared at the psychology department for my orientation and my assignment, ready for whatever I had to do, like it or not. Failure was not an option. My indoctrination and job-launching interview at the psych department included agreeing to work under a professor in an area in which I had absolutely *no* interest, and working under someone whom I didn't much care for either (I didn't tell him that, of course). But I had already said yes to my admission and the conditions of my sentence. This was the other side of the spent coin. I couldn't and wouldn't ask for it back. You know, I had jumped in. The boat now speeding off, it was ride, sink, or swim.

Forced voluntarily to enroll in two graduate psychology courses, as well as an undergraduate Intro to Psych class since I had never had a psychology course, I had little standing to object. I signed up. I belonged to them, and psychology as a whole. But my life was pretty much a mess, so what did I have to lose? I remember being warned sternly that I must be the top student in that 350-student Intro Psych class, or I would be removed from the grad program!

I had to work harder to do well and be the top student in that Intro Psych class than just about any graduate psychology course I took thereafter. I had a lot to learn—what we call a steep learning curve. I studied pretty hard, to finish with the second-highest grade in the class. But they didn't give me the boot.

To enhance my ability to read volumes of psychology textbooks in rapid "catch-up" mode, I decided to take a course in speed-reading. That should help, right? Unfortunately, it was only later that I found a great description of speed-reading from Woody Allen: "I took a course in speed-reading and was able to read *War and Peace* in 20 minutes. It's about Russia."

That was pretty much the result of my trying to become a better student and reader through warp speed-reading. It didn't work (surprise!), and it almost ruined my love of reading. Come to think of it, graduate school nearly had the *same* effect. But I'm preaching to the choir for all you graduate student types. Have *you* ever taken a speed-reading course? If so, you know what I'm talking about. If not, don't. But I pressed on, and being a medium-slow reader, I persevered.

I felt the pressure to perform academically in a way I never had before. Then, as a barely passing graduate student, I found myself incredibly drawn into the world of child psychology and the hospital setting—two colliding spheres that went on to define my next several years.

Child Psychology?

My initial learning—slow reading—about psychology occurred as a master's-level graduate student, and especially during my time working in a children's hospital. This was before I made the jump to the *dark side* and entered the doctoral program in clinical psychology, and it certainly played a critical role in my learning and humbling preparation for a life as an adult psychologist, teacher (especially), therapist, professor, and even researcher. It was mostly a good period in my early career and life, but not entirely so—though it was always interesting and sometimes even entertaining.

I never wanted to be a child psychologist, but like so much of my psychology journey, I pretty much fell into it—that deep dark pit of crazy kid behavior and brat attack. But after a while, it kind of grew on me—not like moss on the north face of an old tree, but more like a peace treaty between warring sides. You'll see what I mean.

Child Psychologist Extraordinaire?

I first fell into it, then willingly threw my hat in to the child arena, finally running for the doors into adult psychology—maybe not screaming, but briskly for sure. To be honest, not all of my child psychologist-ness went so wrong, and it was a good place to start. Here are how my adventures in child psychology went.

You might say I spent three powerful years lateral learning—first in speech pathology, and then in special education and at a wonderful children's hospital. My invite into the field of speech pathology came about when a professor from that department and school approached my major professor in the experimental psych master's program in which I was enrolled.

Their department was looking for help with a multiply handicapped girl in their speech clinic who needed to learn to use her fingers for sign language—leading us to invent a kind of biofeedback device and method. It was a fascinating problem. She had cerebral palsy (CP), a severe physical disability from brain damage at birth, and was functionally deaf and mute. Blanca (which means "white" or by extension "pure" in Spanish—an appropriate descriptor for this pretty, sweet child) couldn't hear or speak. Her parents were told by various professionals, physicians primarily, that this completely uncommunicative child was profoundly "retarded" (an old term we don't use anymore) and should be institutionalized. Her loving and wise parents said, "No, she is smart—look at her eyes." They were actually bright and attentive, I thought, suggesting intelligence beneath her intensely crooked smile and spastic head and arm movements.

Standardized intelligence tests are near useless with a severely physically disabled, deaf, and mute child. But that didn't stop the brilliant experts from employing them, declaring her profoundly mentally retarded and "unrehabilitatable" (I think I invented this word) or ever teachable. When the parents finally and providentially made their way to the university speech clinic 10 years later, a special nonverbal IQ test was finally and appropriately employed and concluded she was of normal intelligence! Outstanding! I think the parents must have wept when they got that final confirmation. I wish I could have been there. Now the problem became how to help her communicate. Sign language!

Amazingly, she learned something like 300 signs in just a few weeks, but soon came up against a wall when finger spelling was required. A severe athetoid/spastic CP like her does not have very good (or any) of the finger dexterity necessary for letter-by-letter spelling of words. So knowing they were overmatched, Blanca and her parents made the short trek from the speech building over to the psych building—where my professor and I were searching for a research project. Voilà!

I fell in love with this sweet 10-year-old Mexican American girl, and *she* became my master's thesis. So I created this very crude biofeedback device—a black metal box with four little lights in a row and a big bulb at the top, all attached to guitar finger picks wired to a battery and the lights (see picture). Crazy. For sure, I was now not only a psychologist-to-be but also a brilliant inventor of a new biofeedback device. Truth be told, I used my father's radio station engineers to help me devise and put together that crude but wonderful mechanism. It's one of my favorite pictures.

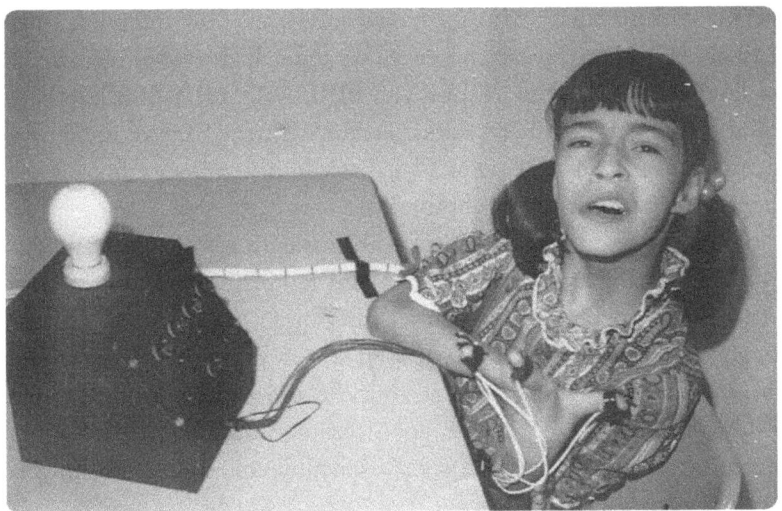

Biofeedback machine in hand (pun intended), I embarked on my plan to teach her the digital task of touching each of her fingers to her thumb (pick) while seeing the lights illuminate with each successive touch. It's a simple task you can do. Try it: touch your index finger to thumb, middle finger to thumb, ring finger to thumb, and little finger to thumb. Probably takes you one to two seconds to complete. It took Blanca 34 seconds to do that *once* during baseline (no light) trials!

The lights were to be her feedback and reinforcement. I added lots of verbal praise each time she made the correct touch in the finger dexterity task. Besides the primary motor disability, CP is also known to have a decrement in proprioceptive awareness of where body parts such as fingers are in space. It was a double whammy! She needed extra help in knowing when her fingers actually touched the thumb. So we pulled out the "big guns" to help—the giant light bulb (you see it on the picture).

But very early in our training, we had this funny (not so much for her) thing happen, confirming my own brilliant, enhanced biofeedback touch (or blow). The fifth light—the big light bulb on the top of the box—was reserved to give a big reward for completing the four-touch task. I found out that was not such a good idea for a person with spasticity and hyperreactive reflexes. Can you guess why? I disabled it after one trial when I just about had to peel her off the ceiling when ALL HER REFLEXES FIRED AT ONCE! (Oops.) It's kind of the way spasticity works. Fortunately, she forgave me after I gently coaxed and then helped her back into her chair from off the floor. One trial learning for both of us.

Amazingly, my thesis project with this enthusiastic, beautiful girl worked like a charm. Our feedback and reinforcement training with the lights (sans big light bulb) decreased her time to touch the four fingers to her thumb from 34 second to 4.5 seconds. It took several weeks and many reinforced trials, but she and we did it! I believe she is now a functional adult with good communication skills, including being able (probably with some difficulty, of course) to finger-spell words.

I wrote up the findings for this research project for publication with my thesis advisor professor, and it was accepted for publication in *The Journal of Nervous and Mental Disease*[1]. It was my first publication, the spotlight of "fame" took hold and I was off to the races of research fame and glory. Yeah, right.

Road to the Hospital Child Psychologist
As a result of this first success in my master's research project, I was invited to take a position at the hospital for multiply handicapped children and adolescents an hour's drive away, while at the same time joining the speech department to study for a master's in speech pathology. So up for the double challenge after such a positive experience with our research with severely handicapped Blanca, I did both.

The Hospital and the Screamer
Can you fall in love with a hospital? Maybe not, but I did.

The hospital was built back in the 1930s to serve the most severely sick and handicapped children, especially those with polio, as well as our polio-stricken president. That made sense, what with its natural hot springs mineral water bubbling up to the indoor and outdoor rehab pools. Adding to its beauty was an elegant courtyard in the center, with a fountain and walls inside and out of bright white everywhere, and a second floor where I lived for three years—free room and board and a living allowance of $300 a month. It worked for me back then.

The town was a curious one and I liked it. It was a smallish western town, just north of the famous fields of green chili America eats and a million-tree pecan grove. It was nestled underneath an older rounded mountain range and national wilderness area with a funny name visitors could never pronounce right, and at the foot of a manmade desert lake named after an elephant. It was strange, what with the big butte rock structure sticking out in its middle that seemed artistically molded by God, with help of course from some volcanic activity. It actually did resemble that elephant's head with the huge African style (not the smaller Indian) floppy ear and likeness of a trunk undulating forward.

It was this setting that ultimately lured me into the world of clinical child psychology. Frankly, it was a crazy welcome, beginning in a semi-appropriate way with screams. No, not mine, but they could and probably should have been.

The screams bombarded their way down to the "special behavior program" teacher. That, of course, was me. And they seemed to be intensifying. Will SOMEBODY PLEASE DO SOMETHING? WAS SOMEONE DYING OR WHAT? I decided I'd better get down there and see what it was all about.

I'd never heard a banshee shriek, and I didn't even know what one was, but it was probably like that. The whole hospital must have heard it, startling me from a walk to a brisk near run in that direction from my spartan little special ed classroom and speech and language therapy room.

Rounding the corner toward the medical ward it was reverberating from, I saw the both terrorized and it turned out terrorizing gaggle of hospital staff who had circled around a boy's bedside. The boy was about 10 with very good lungs and a vocal apparatus to match. You know that shriek that babies can make when they are demanding attention or registering alarm? Like that. He loudly warned them, "DO NOT TOUCH ME."

The hospital cadre included nurses, of course, and PTs (physical therapists—better known as "physical terrorists" by those they abuse), along with other ward staff. And then there was me, with my couple of student assistants in tow close behind. When I appeared, they all turned their heads and gave me that look: "What the h--- are *you* doing here? Can't you see we are busy?" and some fearful faces seemed to add the second look: "Please help. Can you take over?"

So this was my accidental introduction to child clinical psychology. It was also my first of many professional interactions with nurses—the ones who actually run the hospitals. These were indeed deep and "dangerous" psychological waters into which I ignorantly jumped. Though an expert swimmer, I didn't know how to swim or even tread those waters. I remember a person telling a friend what it was like to be overwhelmed with stressful incompetence when being asked to take on a new high-demand project—an extra kid. He responded: "Imagine you are drowning, there is no one there to save you, and someone hands you a baby." Got it. That was me.

But what happened next shocked everyone there, including me, and ultimately ignited a career I'm going to tell you all about.

Clearly, our 10-year-old screamer, who was post-op for knee surgery and clearly in pain, was not happy. So, I guess it would have to be behavior modification guy to the "rescue." I knew how to train dogs (and certainly not cats), so how could it be any harder than that?

The boy was screaming murder each time a physical terrorist, I mean therapist, went near him to "range" (flex, or "torture"—you choose the term) his leg and knee in the split cast of the just-operated-on leg. It was no doubt excruciatingly painful, but the PTs were under doctor's orders to range (again, "torture") his leg so it wouldn't go into a fixed contracture and he could never walk on it. I think they tried it once, when they forcibly bent his leg, and only once. He wouldn't let them near him after that. With nods of reluctant permission from the PTs and now traumatized nurses as well, I asked if I could help, and all of a sudden, the case was mine.

Thinking a bit—something I was trained to do some time ago in school—I asked one PT to get me a goniometer, which measures angles in degrees, to tape at the split-cast knee joint, so as to measure the angle of knee flexion. The boy was still crying when I moved in for the "kill," I mean behavioral treatment, while promising effusively not to touch him or force him to move his leg or knee. The PTs and my students curiously stood by, along with the ward nurses. "Let's see how this fool Mr. Behaviorist will do."

I explained to the boy that I was going to let him decide whether and how much he was going to bend his knee, if at all, standing back a distance enough from him that he knew I wasn't going to touch him. At this point, the PTs under those doctor's orders were thinking, "We are going to trust this idiot to do our work and then we are going to get in trouble for not ranging his knee?" But they held back to see.

I asked the boy if he could show me how far he could bend his knee without any pain. The looks I got from the PTs and nurses, and probably my students, were similar to what you would see when you told people you were going to grow a third arm right before them. But

I knew that a good chunk of pain is from the psychological suffering side, and not just the physiological sensation (that's called, should you be interested, "nociception"—you will be tested on that at the end of the tour).

With some coaxing, by a miracle, the boy stopped crying and said he couldn't do it. The negotiation was on. I told him to try anyway so we could see. He did, mainly to prove me wrong, but there occurred a nearly imperceptible movement—maybe a half a degree (that is a *very small* movement). So I shocked everyone, including him, when I immediately cheered and praised him loudly for doing such a great job. "You did it!" When I asked him to try again and see if he could beat that amazing record, he reluctantly did, probably got to a whole degree of flexion. My cheering and praise were picked up by the students who chimed in, and then the PTs and nurses, as we continued.

Would you believe that the boy got up to a 45-degree flexion, on his own, without crying out in pain or being touched or "ranged" by anyone. He was in control. There were cheers all the way around, and from this little episode he is probably walking today *and* (most importantly) my fame spread throughout the hospital and pretty much citywide! (I'm lying about the city fame. But it could have. It was a small city.)

Speech Pathology and Special Ed to Clinical Psychology

While completing my master's in speech pathology as I continued to work and live at the children's hospital, I played dual roles: speech and language and special education teacher—and budding child psychologist/behavior modifier. As it turned out, I stayed on the new path to clinical psychology, but not abandoning speech pathology just yet—she was not done with me.

Certainly, this was not because the field of speech pathology is about 95 percent beautiful women. That shouldn't influence this serious student of psychology. I once attended their ASHA Convention in Detroit as a wild bachelor, and I came very close to saying goodbye to psychology and pursuing speech pathology for some other very valid reason that I can't exactly recall at the moment.

I was now approaching becoming a professional student, according to my father's thinking. He once attempted to question my dual school and work life, but it turned into a blessing. He told me he knew why I stayed in school so long (I was fully expecting a put-down for being afraid to come out into the real world like him): "Because you love to learn." I guess he was right. But there was much more learning to come!

While in speech pathology school, during my lateral learning curve climb, I decided to take two most interesting classes: Sign Language and Stuttering. There was fun and craziness in both. The first interest you can figure out had to do with my wonderful time with Blanca. But the second? I'll get to that.

Like Blanca, I found that I, too, was not so good at sign language or finger spelling, though I had no excuse of physical disability. Indeed, if you can believe this, I was a sign language STUTTERER. Two speech disabilities in one! It must have been a record of sorts! Interestingly, our exam in that class was to give a speech in front of the class and professor, totally in sign language and finger spelling. No talking. In front, I froze. Blanca likely would have done a better job than I did, even in the finger spelling. Imagine a stuttering, shaky, jittery fingering speller, with stops and extraneous movements, etc., just like a bad stutterer. That was me. Funny. I think I passed that class, embarrassment and all.

My stuttering class was even more fascinating. We had to learn about what the stutterer experiences and were required to mimic it. The final exam (or one of the exams or tasks, I forget) had to do with going out in the community in pairs and stuttering in front of others, say in a store or restaurant. One stuttered, and the other observed and took notes, to return to a meeting where we all shared our experience. By the way, I got very good at stuttering, with head movements and facial grimaces, starts and stops, drawn-out syllables, and stuck-on consonants. I could show off I was so good at it, sort of like when I'd fake a fall down a long stairway, arms flailing, feet rapidly slipping and sliding off each step—landing at the bottom upright, unharmed, smiling.

I performed so well during my "episode," showing off a bit like my false fall down the stairwell, in front of the terrified salesclerk. When people stutter, there are one of three responses they get from others. First, the person (impatient) tries to jump in constantly and finish your words and even sentences. They get impatient and frustrated and just want the darn stutterer to finish! "What do you want???" is the look you are likely to get.

The second responder just runs off, in a panic often, Mr. Bean-like. This might be as soon as he or she recognizes, "Oh no, this person stutters. I've got to get out of here!" This escape is usually rapid and can occur at any point in the attempted stuttering communication. The third is the empathic person, listening and tuning into what the stutterer is trying to say, maybe even mirroring the sounds and gestures of the stutterer, no matter how long and drawn out the "conversation."

I honestly don't know which one is worse. I do know when I really laid on the severe stuttering routine, that I, the stutterer, would take on the anxiety of the person listening. It was a weird thing.

CAN WE TALK?

How to Help a Stutterer. Something to keep in mind when faced with a bad stutterer: most importantly, listen. Wait, don't rush off or rush the person. You will make it worse for both of you. I learned to have a good enough ear for the different types of stuttering, the therapies that can work, what probably won't, and what can make it worse. Yes, it's a condition that is related to anxiety, but the lion's share of the anxiety is more likely the *result* of the stuttering and not necessarily the *cause* of the stuttering. It is more complicated than that, and there are many theories about what causes it.

We know *every* kid goes through a period in which they stutter. It's a normal part of learning to speak. They are learning language and expression and will often rush into talking before their thoughts are formed fully. Hey, we adults do this too! It's normal for a five- or six-year-old to do this, but not so much for an eight- or nine-year-old. Leave them alone and if they are still stuttering by about eight, then consider therapy with a speech therapist or speech pathologist (the formal term). There are lots of good ones—therapies and speech therapists. But don't force them into psychological therapy—that is unless there are some pretty good reasons to believe their childhood experiences (trauma?) are related to an anxiety state that can produce or worsen stuttering.

My training and practice in speech pathology taught me to discriminate their type of stuttering, along with other speech impediments like lisps, as well as what therapy the stutterer or person misarticulating had received. For example, by how he or she pushed or slid through the various stops and catches, or positioned their tongues and lips in malforming words and sounds.

One interesting therapy for stuttering is called delayed auditory feedback, or DAF. Did you know that if you play back what stutterers are saying, about a half a second after they speak, that it will force the person to slow down and extend each word and sound. It's the only way you can talk during DAF. It can help you not stutter if you are a stutterer but *make* you a stutter if you aren't one already. If you are ever able to get hooked up to DAF, you will see (and hear) what I mean. It's weird.

The most fun aspect of our community stuttering abuse exercise happened when we all met at a local bar and sandwich shop to share our stories. But one girl didn't complete the stuttering task in front of others. So the professor decided to enforce the exercise by having her go over to these two men at a separate table and stutter in front of them and then come back and tell us all how it went and what it was like for her. She got up, walked over slowly to the table, addressed the two, and sat down. After about 30 minutes we were wondering what happened. She had sat down and was having a conversation (presumably stuttering) with the two men. Finally, she came back and told us: "You are not going to believe what happened there. They were

BOTH stutterers! So I had to stay and stutter along with them, rather than revealing I was not actually a stutterer so as not to offend them and embarrass me!"

It wasn't long into my time at the hospital for disabled children that I was inevitably drawn into the clinical arena—you might say wonderful "circus"—of child psychology. Before I get into it, though, I want to tell you about a few of the other kids that I ended up working with using psychology and speech and language therapy.

Ella

Delegated to the children's hospital, I was introduced to one of my new speech and language clients, Ella. She was a pretty 10-year-old Navajo girl who could not talk and was diagnosed with cognitive disability (we are not supposed to say "mental retardation" anymore so I won't, but that was her diagnosis at the time). My job was to help her talk and to communicate, and then to teach her things like the "3 Rs." But talking came first. No matter what I tried, she would hardly make a sound. So, I pulled out the "big guns"—M&M candies. For every sound she emitted—some I had to prime by pushing gently on her stomach—I would put an M&M on her tongue, accompanied by praising her verbally. This intervention went on for some weeks, as I kept track of her response rate on my graphs.

When I presented my graph of progress (there wasn't so much) to my supervisor in the speech clinic (I was still completing my master's in speech pathology at this time), he asked me pointedly, "Why are you punishing her?" "Punishing her!" I exclaimed. "I was reinforcing her with M&M's (the universal reinforcer, right?). What kid doesn't love M&M's chocolates?"

Not so fast, John. Pointing out the declining vocalization response rate to the intervention, he asked me: "What is the definition of punishment?" A quiz. Great. I know the answer: "Any stimulus or event paired or associated with a response or behavior that causes the behavior to decrease, or its probability in the future to decrease." By the decreasing responses to my M&M "reinforcement" intervention, I realized—brilliantly, I should add—I had been punishing her! So my professor picked up this paddle—like the kind you get in college from your fraternity—and BEAT ME with it (providing a fine illustration of what punishment really looks and feels like). As I ran screaming from his office, he yelled, "YOU ARE THE MOST USELESS GRADUATE STUDENT I'VE EVER HAD. NOW GET OUT AND NEVER COME BACK, AND YOU CAN FORGET ABOUT EVER GETTING YOUR MASTER'S DEGREE FROM THIS SCHOOL OR ME AS YOUR MAJOR PROFESSOR!"

Now you know that did not happen. But it was fun to imagine, right? Speaking of imagining, I believe that thought crossed my professor's mind, perhaps gleefully, as he glanced at the paddle (actually) hung on his wall—probably for those tougher speech pathology cases that refused to follow therapeutic directions. Nevertheless, an important teachable moment for me. I did manage to stay in school and get my degree under him, somewhat miraculously to be honest.

Not one to admit defeat so easily, I decided to stay with the program with Ella (wisely avoiding the professor for a time) and rethought things about my reinforcement conundrum. Hmmmm. Maybe there would be something other than the M&M's that she would actually like and work to get. Then it came to me: Froot Loops! I had a box of them for some strange reason in my classroom cabinet (probably leftover from the last teacher who fled the scene) and thought why not. So the Froot Loop intervention commenced. And you know what? Ella loved them, made more and more sounds and words to earn more. Reinforcement. Voilà! Success!

But the Ella story had another chapter in my learning to work with kids (and parents). Her parents came in from the Navajo reservation and tribal lands to have a consultation with her doctors and teacher, me. When we met, they were quiet, and I expected such. The Navajos are a proud people of few words, I was told, and learned in time. But I knew I would be able to have a good discussion with them. It was their daughter after all. The interview lasted for about 30 minutes, with the parents who sat across from me, sitting up straight, arms crossed, motionless and expressionless. Oh, there was an expression, but I was not so sure it was positive.

So I did all the talking, not by design, but by necessity. They said not a single word the whole time. I felt somewhat downcast after they left. I had failed to do my job. What a terrible parent conference. When I asked some of my colleagues at the hospital who had a better sense of the Indian culture, I was informed that I probably did nothing wrong. They said that Navajos did not typically speak when they don't have anything important to say, and they obviously didn't. I wish I and some others I know could be more like that; as the Bible says: "Be quick to listen, slow to speak, and slow to anger." But no talk at all? Anyway, I got a window into the nonverbal environment she had grown up in. It was in some real ways a reflection of why I was having such trouble getting sounds from dear Ella, and I don't remember us ever making much progress. She did like all the Froot Loops, however. Unfortunately, they were not my snack of choice.

As a speech and language therapist at the children's hospital, I encountered the opposite from many parents of nonverbal kids, or those with speech impediments. We would sometimes tell a funny story to parents who always talked and did *too much* for their kids, not requiring them to learn to talk. It goes like this: There was a boy who never talked. But he did well in school and seemed otherwise normal. Every specialist the parents took their kid to said the same thing: there is no reason why your son cannot talk. Finally, one day when the now teenaged son was sitting down to breakfast, the mother burned his toast. When she brought the toast to the son, all apologies, he blurted out: "What's the meaning of this?!" The mother broke down crying, hugged her previously nonverbal son, and finally asked him: "Why haven't you talked before now?" His answer: "Everything was fine until now."

One time I had a client who had a very harsh, raspy voice. It was not normal. So we began working together to help him to soften his voice (relaxing his vocal cords, larynx, and neck muscles). At the end of each week at the hospital with me, he would make great progress. But each Monday, after his weekend at home, he'd come back with the same raspy voice. What was up, I wondered. Then I asked for a conference with the parents, and (you guessed it), HIS

FATHER TALKED JUST LIKE THAT, WITH THE HARSH RASPY VOICE! Dad didn't know what was wrong with the way his son talked. I responded with something like, "I think you are right." Therapy over.

IQ—Me

A good part of my job as a special education teacher and speech therapist was to conduct assessments of intellectual functioning and learning. It was not my favorite thing, but I learned some valuable lessons—besides distrusting the standardized tests we are saddled with.

My initial method of getting children to come with me for testing was to ask them: "Do you want to come with me to answer some questions for me?" Guess what these kids would say? You got it: "No." They didn't want to come with me. Why should they? *Then* what do you say or do? Oh, sure, something like, "Well, we are going to do this anyway." Good luck, buddy. I soon learned, lawyer-like, to never ask a question to which I didn't want to hear the answer, or to give a choice when there was none. I learned to say: "Hey, we get to go take some fun tests and do some things together!" No option. Learning on the job.

Time to Leave

I remember the day I decided it was time for me to leave the hospital and seek greater things—adult psychology! Here's what happened: I had been conducting an IQ test on a young five-year-old girl who had been referred for special education for obvious good reasons. But it was one of those occasions when I felt as if I was in the presence of true genius—she was acing most of the questions! This was impossible. She was a special ed student! Nevertheless, my excitement grew as I began assessing her performance and score. I found that she was of *normal intelligence*. I was so used to testing mentally and physically disabled children that I had lost sight of what normal was like. I had *no* idea. So, I decided I wanted to find out what normal adults were like, applied, and got into a doctorate program in clinical psychology with a specialization in adults. I should also admit that an additional motivation was to go get the higher, doctorate degree so I wouldn't have to listen to those pontificating Ph.D. "consultants" the hospital would bring in to "help" me. (Have you ever heard the definition of Ph.D.?—"piled higher and deeper," following in kind after the B.S. and M.S. degrees. You get it, right? Don't tell anyone I told you.)

> **CAN WE TALK?**
>
> IQ.—What does it mean? I'm so glad you asked. (You did, didn't you?) No matter. Now I've got some shots to take at these IQ-believers, as well as the equally weird personality testing folks. In my humorous (not to them!) thinking, I've concluded their IQ-less personality dizziness may have caused them to fall out of the same tree, on their heads. You'll see what I mean. (In a coming Can We Talk? I'll address the related concepts of psychological gullibility, what we call "Barnum statements," and personality diagnosis craziness, so stay tuned)
>
> Okay, IQ or intelligence quotient. I guess we all have one, whether you are tested or not (yes?). Of course, there has to be a single number that can identify your so-called inalterable, absolute intelligence. Really? The folks in my field of psychology who argue that, besides being certifiably lamebrained, believe in the G, or general intelligence. I think these are a rarer and rarer breed of assessment-obsessed psychologists. We can only hope. This has done so much harm to society, kids especially. Did you ever hear the Prairie Home Companion radio program in which Garrison Keillor makes appropriate fun of IQ?—that everyone in that town has above-average intelligence—crazy! There is a black version of an IQ test, poking sarcastic and well-deserved fun at the IQ test in which whites score generally higher than blacks, and there is my little Blanca who couldn't speak or hear and was "found" to have an IQ in the severely mentally retarded range. She was about to be relegated to an institution for the mentally retarded (old words we no longer use), and she was treated as such until she was taught sign language, could finally communicate, and was found to have normal intelligence by an appropriate test for the communication challenged.

> *Important Question:* Is this IQ test a test of learning and experience, or some sort of absolute, innate intelligence that cannot be changed? Did you know that the first so-called intelligence test was the Binet, which was developed in Paris, France to determine learning performance in French students? It was never intended to serve as an inalterable intelligence rating. Then, a smart aleck psychologist from Stanford University (name of this egghead not revealed to protect the guilty) took the Binet, made it into the Stanford-Binet, one of the most widely used intelligence tests for children, and foisted (my favorite word again) it on the rest of us.
>
> *Suggestion:* Pay no attention to the IQ test and especially that absolutely idiotic quotient number (ironies intended). Pay more attention to things like learning, achievement, mastery, wisdom, gifts and giftedness, life skills and strengths, courage, honesty and integrity, humility, faithfulness (godliness?), happiness, love, and service—the enduring qualities or "absolutes." (Look forward to another upcoming Can We Talk? on Gifts and Giftedness, etc., for a further, more intelligent, but IQ-less, discussion on this point.) A person's heart, as well as his or her EQ, or emotional quotient, might be a much more valid and useful characteristic (but watch out when someone tries to put a number on it and judge you by it). Those are the important things. Forget the rest.

Path to the Ph.D.

After finishing my two master's programs, degrees in hand, and time at the children's hospital as a speech therapist and special education teacher, I began to cast my eyes and heart onward—to the yellow brick Ph.D. road.

ROOM 203

WELCOME TO THE DOCTORAL PROGRAM

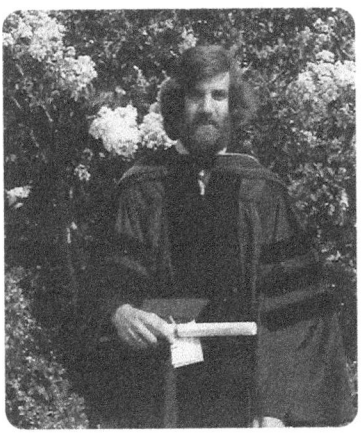

"Remember that a kick in the butt is a step forward."

—UNKNOWN

Even if you have taken multiple psych courses or (oh no) majored in psychology, you probably have not gone so far as to seek an advanced degree in psychology, like a doctorate. But, obviously, I did. Would I do it again if I could turn the clock back, avoid further school and psychological "abuse," and stay at the children's hospital where I'd become so happy?—"Good question!"

Upon arriving at my next university for more of that crazy education necessary for becoming an *actual* psychologist, I was fresh off my time working at the hospital for multiply handicapped children and adolescents with two master's degrees in hand. This is not to mention the arrogance of one who already knew all he needed to know. Just give me the degree, I thought. My attitude was well reflected by my suggestive question to the doctoral program's department head about whether I could finish the doctoral work in a year. The department head professor humored me humorlessly, saying, though unlikely, let's just see. Well, we certainly did, one move across half the country, demolishing my little Toyota meeting a deer at 60 miles per hour in the road at night—the results shown here, deer "impression" on the grill (not really), but nicely dressed for some reason. Either way, a likely bad omen. Should have paid more attention to that, but didn't, and then three intense years later.

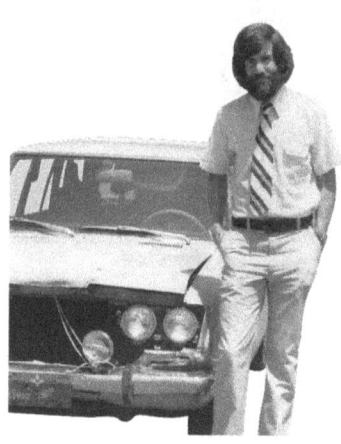

It was the fall of 1974 when I finally arrived on campus for the presumably last leg in my university education, punctuated by my three years at the children's hospital *playing* psychologist. I found that there was a whole class of master's-level students like myself who had been recruited for this doctoral program. It was flush with fellowship and assistantship money from the state of Alabama for our support, a good thing.

Settling into my new life phase and challenges ahead, I was reasonably happy to be there, but not nearly as happy as our fellow new student from Korea. His English wasn't so great, but with "acceptance letter" in hand, he was there all the way from his home country. The problem was, it was not an acceptance letter, but a rejection letter. I don't know if you have ever gotten this kind of a letter, with a long description of your fine qualifications, but at the end came the key sentence saying something like, "however," "unfortunately," or "we regret to inform you."

We felt horrible for him and understood his dilemma. The program could not, would not, send him all the way back home to South Korea with a "so sorry about that. Have a nice day and a good trip home." I was proud of the program. They decided to let him stay and take the standard doctoral courses while on probation for the year, to let him earn his full acceptance for the degree. Sadly, he wasn't able to compete and complete the courses, and so was gone by year's end. I sometimes wonder what happened to him.

My bizarre thinking cap on, I surmised how you could get into a school (or job) from which you were actually rejected. Now this plan is provided to you readers free of charge, and donations will be accepted for successful use of its corrupt "wisdom." Do not try to contact me should you get in trouble for attempting the following:

1. Show up at the school, department, or job site with rejection letter in hand, in old, tattered clothes with a beat-up suitcase and clothes spilling out the sides.
2. Have a bad English accent of some sort (you pick the country), and state that you are from a faraway place, noting that you could only afford a one-way ticket there.
3. Ask where the low-cost housing is (or dorm) so you can go get settled before the first class or day at work.

Further note to reader: Please **do not** *use the above in your effort to sabotage your way into school or a job position. I will renounce ever encouraging or leading you to do that. You are on your own. It was a stupid joke.*

As for me, not requiring steps one through three, though barely getting accepted, I'm sure, I arrived on campus for the start of my doctoral education. Fortunately, I was able to take a position as a resident assistant over a freshman dorm. It was not my best decision. It was crazy. The guys loved aiming fireworks and bottle rockets at my window—hilarity for them, not so much for me. This also was the Bible Belt, and my door was regularly accosted by evangelicals wanting to know if I had been "saved." I told them I was Jewish to dispatch them without a long discourse on religion and Jesus (not true, but what did they know). That got rid of them quickly enough, curiously ironic since I had heard Jesus was a Jew.

Before getting to be a teacher and professor, I had to first crawl the student gauntlet through various doctoral-level graduate instructors and professors. That began during my two master's degree programs and then again in the much more perfected, and in many ways more nefarious, doctoral program teaching experiences and professional hazing. I was a graduate student subjected to the same kind of teaching weirdness I later administered to those students with the unfortunate karma to have fallen under my professorial thumb. Hey, I got "teaching crazed," why not pass it on—my karma, their karma, sheer meanness, and probably a combination of them all.

My least favorite class we all were required (read: abusively forced) to take was experimental statistics—not my glass of beer. I was pretty sure I was a right-brain guy in that left-brain world of academic psychology and science. I think I received the lowest B grade (a B-----...) ever given, and that was even a gift. We all knew, and were reminded periodically, that a "C" in graduate school is a failing grade. Take the course over (with permission) if you are lucky, get put on probation, or be expelled from the program. Some choice.

I remember sitting in one of those doctoral-level stat classes trying to figure out what in the world this new professor was talking about. He had a curious (read: irritating) habit of rapidly writing formulas across the wall of blackboards at the front of the classroom while talking into the board (no, not to himself, though in a real way he was), as we foolish students struggled to keep up writing all those unintelligible formulas. Only then, at the end of the board, would he pause, scratch, and shake his head, and *furiously erase all the formulas with his tie*—a white chalky sleet (yes, sleet) storm dusting him and the two front rows of previously attentive students.

I found out later, to my great ire, that the grad students who did best on the exams and, ultimately, the course, *never came to class!* It was explained to me when I demanded an answer from those slackers that the prof confused them all so much, it was better not to go but to read the chapters and meet with study groups. "NOW you tell me!" I disgustedly replied.

One semester in the stat course series, this same poor professor announced that over the last two weeks of class, we would be going through four big chapters (maybe 150 pages of formulas!). Say what?

He was kidding, for sure. Nope, dead serious. Determined to learn enough to get through the course, I decided I was just going to raise my hand each time I didn't understand something and ask for him to explain. So I did, ultimately to his great consternation. At first, he would call on me, attempt to answer my well-formed question, and explain what he meant, then turn back to the board and resume his furious formula writing. Not having ANY idea of what he said or meant, I raised my hand almost immediately once again.

This river dance (or wrestling match) went on, sans music, for a decent portion of the class, until I just KEPT my hand up for the whole class—Moses holding his war staff skyward at the battle plain (yet with no Aaron or Jethro to help hold it up)—staring darts at him in his retreat to the faceless blackboard until class was over. I was rude, and mad. I complained to the chairman of the department after a couple of these arm-sore classes and was informed that he was a new professor and just learning to teach, so bear with him. WHAT? Bear with him? It was a grace I needed later in my learning to teach, so in retrospect I should have been kinder to him (*and* to the future me).

As I've mentioned, I entered the doctoral program with a group of other master's-level "know-it-alls." We were radical behaviorists, meaning we believed in behavior exclusively—dismissing the "black box" between stimulus, response, and consequence. No mind, belief, spirit (please, no!), or even thoughts were important enough for our attention. Mind you (oops), this was before cognitive psychology or cognitive behavioral therapy (CBT) came into their own. It was the psychoanalysts vs. the behaviorists (I'm ignoring the client-centered modalities—Carl Rogers and Bill (WR) Miller will forgive me). We were the roosters (I'm refraining from using the actual term here) ruling the roost of psychology—at least in our own minds (oops again, I mean behavior).

We loved and followed the learning theorists and psychologists who were considered radical behaviorists (like our hero B.F. Skinner) and were not well accepted by the more eclectic students and professors. Go figure. We loved to also irritate the teachers, especially the more traditionalist and psychodynamic ones—like the goofy believers and promoters of projective testing.

My anti-testing bias (I mean well-founded belief) was further radicalized, we might say, in my doctoral training during the psychodynamic/projective testing block of courses. One time I was thrown out of class—along with other "radical" behaviorist students—for poking some well-deserved fun at those strange (and generally unvalidated) tests like the Draw-a-Person, the House-Tree-Person, and the Mt. Olympus of all projectives, the Rorschach inkblot test. Horrors!

One especially hilarious memory was when a buddy decided to complete one of his tests that the client failed to complete, by drawing it in himself—as a man standing, feet apart, with his hands on his hips. When asked by the very thoughtful and pensive professor what the class and he thought that meant, he finally blurted out: "Offsides?" (For you non-sports types, that is the signal from the referee that the football player is offsides, and his team will be penalized five yards.) Despite the fact that it was quite funny, and I'm thinking the whole class, but not the professor, laughed, my behaviorist buddy (Bruce M.) was unfairly and humorlessly thrown out! The rest of us followed shortly. No sense of humor in these (especially projective) test people. What are you going to do?

Child Psychologist without the Child
During my training in the clinical therapy aspect of psychology, we were lectured by a well-known "child psychologist." I use the term child psychologist with reservations, since he didn't much like dealing with kids. That's probably not true, but it could have been. He described his approach to problem kids who were referred to him for help—either by another therapist or professional in the field, or by their very own distraught parents:

He first asked to see the parents, not the kid. WHAT? "It's our kid who has the problem, NOT US," the parents would complain vigorously on the initial phone interview with him. Yep. Not interested in the kid so much. So the parents would drag their reluctant rear ends into the "shame zone," no doubt to be confronted with how it was all their fault for their child's evil ways. But not so fast. He was smarter than to do that, even though it was mostly true. His first assignment, without learning all that much about the kid's horrible behaviors, was for the parents to track and record all the kid's *positive* behavior. "But he/she never does anything good!" was the typical retort. Nevertheless, they dutifully complied. They knew this would be easy since there wasn't much to record. Nothing, for instance.

But a week later, the parents returned with shocked looks. Both had written a veritable book on the kid's positive behaviors. They had *no* idea about all the good things their child did! The wise child psychologist then gave them another assignment. "Now, begin to praise your child each time he/she does one of those good things." So they did, and wouldn't you know the positive behavior increased so much—crowding out the negative behavior opportunities—that no more therapy was needed, and certainly not for their now wonderful kid!

This so-called child psychologist shared another story. He was working with a kid in a classroom situation (yes, sometimes he did directly do child psychology). He implemented praise for quiet, attentive, or studious behavior. But each time he noticed those behaviors and he approached the child to give praise, the kid *stopped* being good and became disruptive and inattentive. After some thought and a bit of behavior data analysis, he recognized that *he* (the psychologist) was not a reinforcer for good behavior, but a punisher. The kid for some reason did not like him. So, brilliantly, he switched his method: whenever the kid was doing something positive, he backed away, and when he was not behaving positively, he approached him. Success! I *loved* this guy. Except for the child thing, I wanted to be like him.

But my path away from kid stuff led to an adult psych primary professor or mentor. I found a good one—or so I thought.

Finding a Mentor

Early in my arrival at the doctoral program, I was attracted to the one new professor as a potential mentor and thesis advisor—

especially because of my past at the children's hospital and that crude biofeedback study I'd completed and published for my psychology master's thesis. He was, for want of a better term at the time, a "medical psychologist." It was a strange newer specialty, and I was warned by other professors I interviewed to find out who best to work under, *not* to choose him because what he did was "not psychology." I was intrigued, and not being one to follow directions or orders, I went to see him. He agreed to have me as one of his six doctoral students. His chosen field without name morphed into the later-birthed fields of behavioral medicine and health psychology—which became my eventual career focus and specialization.

My professor was a brilliant teacher and researcher, and I was soon engaged in projects he chose. He said he didn't care how I did in my classes, but only what research I was involved in and what publications we could get. He noted more than once to each of us six or so students under him that no one would ever ask you what grades you got in graduate school (turned out to be true), but would ask about what research you did and how many publications you were listed on as an author. You've probably heard what you call the person who just barely graduated from medical school with minimally passing grades: "Doctor."

I remember a conversation my mentor had with my father, who had come to visit some time after my doctoral graduation. When my dad asked this professor if I was his best student, my professor/mentor said "No." What? I was shocked. Though he continued: "But he has been my most successful student." (Apologies to my fellow doc students. He was probably lying because my dad was there.) But saved by the bell. My father still thought I was too afraid of the world and not smart enough to make it on my own, in business such as he had. Looking back, I'm thinking—not a bad career if you can get it. (I would later counsel my doctoral students and clinical interns who wanted a career like mine, that mine was not available to them. I wasn't giving it up anytime soon.)

My latter student days were not all fun and games. I worked hard to skip a year or two, because of my master's courses and double degrees, by challenging courses and passing their exams. But not so fast, John. The research we grad students were required to participate in included being plugged into projects under the professor and usually included programming electronics in the laboratory. Not one of my strong suits. One late night, our dig-a-bit pre-computer wiring setup and programming broke down and I had to call and wake him for help. Not happy, he stormed into the lab, looked briefly at the mess of programming wires, flipped one switch, gave us the "you idiot" look, turned and left—and it all returned suddenly and miraculously to proper functioning. Shamed.

I once read about the story of Henry Ford and the notable physicist Steinmetz, who had invented the great turbines that ran Ford's 1920 auto assembly line. One day, the turbines broke down and Ford Motor Co. was losing millions of dollars a day with the stopping of all production. Ford summoned Steinmetz to come and fix them, no matter the cost. Steinmetz did, and the production line came back to life. Steinmetz sent a bill to Ford for $10,000 (remember these were 1920 dollars, worth far more than today's). Ford hit the ceiling! It was an outrageous amount—especially since Ford learned from his supervisors that Steinmetz spent only about ten minutes "fiddling" and then threw some switches and got it all working. Ford demanded an itemized bill. Steinmetz broke the bill down as such: Charge for 10 minutes of fiddling: $100. Charge for knowing where and how to fiddle: $9,900. Ford paid the bill.

My professor knew both where and how to fiddle, and how to trap unsuspecting students, like me. Once, he stashed a cigarette butt on the lab floor in a special place—using the marked item technique—to check to see if we were sweeping the lab as required in one of our duties. When we swore we had been keeping the lab clean, sweeping every day, he calmly pointed out the cigarette still in its place, undisturbed. Caught!

I can't say he was kind about our infractions and imperfections either, and he wasn't always the most encouraging professor and mentor, but he got the most out of us. For me at least, that's what it took. I remember a particular phase of emotional and physical exhaustion, when I was at the virtual end of my rope. He let me have it over something or other. It didn't matter what. He reminded me sometimes of my verbally abusive father. I reacted traumatically, broke down crying, and yelled back at him. It was something I'd wanted, but was always afraid to do, with my father. Suffice to say, it's something you'd generally never do to your holding-all-the-cards professor and thesis advisor. Fortunately, realizing I was about to quit school and working with him, he calmed down and administered enough positives to draw me back in. He did have empathy, just not as much as we needed or wanted back from him.

Clinical Supervision
Being mentored in graduate school in clinical psychology also included clinical supervision in working with clients—learning how to do therapy. But my mentor's direct style sometimes required my skin to be thicker than humanly possible—and I was too thin-skinned as it was. I guess it was what I needed. He never minced words, though many times they had the sting of hurtful criticism and put-downs. Here's an example I remember well.

I was seeing a woman in the training clinic and I came to him for help when I noticed she was not doing her homework or adhering to other parts of the therapy. I showed him her data and he commented: "Why do you keep advising her and giving her new strategies to do?" I answered weakly to his irritated reaction, noting that when she came in without having followed my instructions, I would modify or weaken them enough so that she might be able to complete them. Then came his figurative slap upside of my psychological head: "She is *not* under your instructional control, so *why* do you keep trying to instruct her?" Hmmm, good question (I didn't dare say that). But this is a typical thing that happens when your clients for some reason do not adhere to instructions in your effort to help them change and problem solve. It requires a more strategic plan for behavioral change, not just more instructions.

So, with his help, I developed a behavioral intervention to help this client change with the use of reinforcement strategies rather than mere telling. But there were two big problems with my behavioral approach. First, it was a time before motivation science and motivational interviewing were known or in the literature, and stages of change and CBT were still in their infancy. We wrongly figured that a person was either motivated and ready to change or not—a binary, black-or-white situation—and there was little or nothing you could do to change a person if you were not in control over his or her reinforcement (rewards) or punishment contingencies and events.

The second big problem: my total ignorance. This was the client who was struggling with terrifying, obsessive thoughts of harming her new and first baby, and the traumatic anxiety, avoidant behavior, and depression that accompanied that terrible stress for having to care totally for a new helpless member of the family for whom she was totally responsible.

But unknown to me, she had *postpartum depression!* She was so hyper aroused, especially around her new baby, she couldn't sleep, was highly emotional, and unable to think clearly and rationally. It was hormonal! And that's mainly why our behavioral and attempt at cognitive and motivational intervention didn't work.

I'd like to say that we referred her for appropriate medical treatment, but this was before her condition was widely understood and its treatment was still in its infancy. We now know that worldwide, roughly 20 percent of all first-time mothers experience significant postpartum depression, and there are excellent therapeutics, including antidepressant medications and hormone treatments widely available.

The *Big* Contract
Then, at the end of my doctoral studies, I dodged an exceptionally large caliber bullet—invoking the equally large caliber *contract* that saved my skin and future career. I'd say it was one of my most significant learning experiences as an advanced doctoral student and it had to do with the dissertation—specifically required for one's doctorate in psychology as an independent research study. It was a story that really happened and has delighted all the people with whom I've shared it, including a whole department of laughing colleagues

during one administrative meeting much later. May I share it? Okay, here goes.

About three-quarters of a year before I was due to be finished, having completed all my coursework, my professor informed me that he was taking another university position and would be leaving. Soon. He made it clear that if I was not completely done conducting my research project, data analysis, written thesis, oral exam and all, he was not coming back to sponsor me or help me graduate. I would have to START ALL OVER with a new professor, project, and all. Years more.

I fearfully developed, approved, and started two or three projects, one of which looked promising to begin collecting data in the lab, in my effort to come up with that acceptable (to him) independent doctoral research thesis. When I finally settled on the one that looked like it could fulfill the requirements, I threw myself in headfirst. I finished setting up the lab, getting approval for the study, recruiting and running the subjects with the help of a couple of great undergrad student assistants given to me, and the data analysis was done. NOW to write it up. Simple, right? No.

I didn't calculate one important thing. I had to write up the study, and I got the worst writer's block and could barely write a word! I didn't know what to do. I saw my future career as a psychologist passing before me quickly.

Having learned enough about behavior change in my learning courses, clinical experiences, and practicum in the doctoral program, I set up a behavior modification intervention *on myself*. I created a written contract that included the harshest kind of punishment for noncompliance I could think of. Now, of course, I knew that reinforcement contracts are always best for creating and maintaining behavior change over the long haul, but I needed drastic and immediate change. Powerful punishment was the ticket.

With that said, I needed someone who would administer the punishment if I failed to write. Now if I was the one to self-administer the aversive consequence, you can guess what would happen. I wouldn't do it. The person I found needed to both be willing to help, a friend perhaps, and have a real mean streak—a willingness to do harm to another without conscience. Murray! He was my buddy, but I thought he could fit the bill. And he did, to my great chagrin.

My contract with Murray required me to produce at least 20 new typed pages of the doctoral thesis every two weeks. If I did *not* produce the typed 20 pages at a certain time and place, then Murray would drop one of three stamped addressed envelopes into the mailbox, containing a check from me for a larger amount than I could afford on my meager graduate assistant salary—written to one of my three most hated organizations: the American Nazi Party, the Ku Klux Klan, and (my apologies to my great colleagues on the other side of the M.D./Ph.D. great wall), the American Psychiatric Association. What made matters worse was that I included an effusively positive letter stating I supported everything they stood for and wanted to be listed as a lifetime donor! Ouch.

Then came the night before the first contracted 20-pager was due. It was a Sunday, and Monday noon was the deadline. I hadn't written or typed a WORD. I called Murray and begged him to give me an extension, PLEASE. I'll never forget that laugh. He uttered the most heinous evil-sounding cackle you could ever imagine. He then informed me what mailbox he was going to be standing next to the next day, with the first check and letter in his hot little hand. I knew then he was serious. I got to work and typed all night, made the 20-page contract, rushed to the Monday mailbox and, I think to his disappointment, exchanged the bloodstained 20-page manuscript for the evil letter. The next two contracts were complied with, I got to tear up all three checks and letters, finished and submitted the dissertation, passed my orals (phew), and even published it in a major scientific journal[2]. More fame to come! Thank you, Murray, my evil friend.

Writing School
When not bound up in fearful writer's block, my mentor taught me to write. Well, he didn't so much teach me as he forced me to do it much better, kicking me to the academic curb with some abusive feedback (what we call "constructive" criticism when we are playing "nice").

CAN WE TALK?

Constructive Criticism. Did you know there is no such thing? There isn't. Any form of criticism is destructive, either to the person or to the goal of "helping" people change. It's literally never constructive or helpful. My demanding father was a pro at "constructive" criticism, and we kids were his victims. Know what I mean? Have you ever heard people say to you that they are "confronting you with love"? Religious people can do this too much, especially when misquoting and wrongly interpreting the Bible. But confrontation is still criticism, especially to the receiver, no matter the "motive." And it still backfires.

Now feedback without criticism (is that possible?) is another thing. I learned some time ago in studying and then teaching and applying motivational counseling, that feedback can be corrective without correcting or criticizing. You can express concern and suggest alternative behaviors without criticizing. It's difficult, but possible. The Bible says to confront with love—a hard combination to carry out indeed. "Confront" here really means to gently and humbly admonish, express concern, and possibly with a loving willingness to help the person, to talk about it. There is an art, science, *and* spirit to it, and how to do it well.

Suggestion: Hang out with people, especially friends, who can help you change without criticizing you—or get therapy from someone who is good at that.

By the way, John Gottman's distinguished 50-plus-year career as a psychologist and professor investigating and working with couples has defined criticism as one of the most harmful and toxic attributes of communication and relationship breakdown and destruction (he refers to it as one of the couple's/relationship's "Four Horsemen of the Apocalypse." The others are defensiveness, withdrawal/stonewalling, and contempt).

Therapy Hint: Find someone to help you stop doing this—criticizing. And find a friend or therapist who never does this. As for you, don't tell me you never criticize. Of course you do. It takes hard work, but you can learn

> and practice noncritical ways of requesting change or at least expressing concern and opening a truly constructive dialogue that majors in listening and caring, and minors in telling.

This critical, teachable moment occurred when I met with him to go over a study I had written up and handed to him previously. I was met with mean-dad-abuser. The paper was scarred with red ink and unkind comments about my terrible writing. I seem to remember sitting there in the hot seat by his desk, and he throwing the "bloody" paper on the floor and stamping on it, uttering something like: "This is garbage, horrible…the worst writing I've ever seen!" I was devastated, went home with my psych tail tucked, having decided to quit school. I'd had it with him, and psychology. I wondered if the merchant Marine was still looking for crew, or if the AmeriCorps offer to work with the Northwest Indian tribes was still active. I believe I wept bitterly too.

The next day, I got back up off the humiliation ground, summoning that anger deep down (probably toward my actual dad), and decided I wasn't going to take it from him. I set up a meeting and marched angrily to his office, demanding a second chance at it and him. That's when grace and wisdom struck. I insisted he tell me how to fix the paper, and he did what I never forgot, and have passed on (not the stamping on poor writing) to many students who came after. He said, "Tell me about the study, what the research to date showed, what your experimental question was, what method you employed, the measures you took, your analysis and results, interpretation, and the overall significance in light of other studies"—or something quite similar.

So I did. About five minutes later, I finished the telling and looked up at him. "Now go write *that*," he said matter-of-factly. I believe I responded, light bulb furiously blinking in my head, with: "Do you mean that good writing is the same as good speaking?" Yes.

This episode on writing abuse and wisdom changed my writing from then on, not to mention my decision to not leave psychology.

It was a lesson (pretty) well learned. It's one of those wisdoms that my horde of future, especially grad, students might be thanking me for as their budding careers in psychology unfold. For me, this was another notch in the path to becoming a simplifier, away from the complications I once thought were indicators of good psychological writing, and ultimately teaching, and psychology in general.

ROOM 204

PSYCHOLOGY TEACHING TRIALS

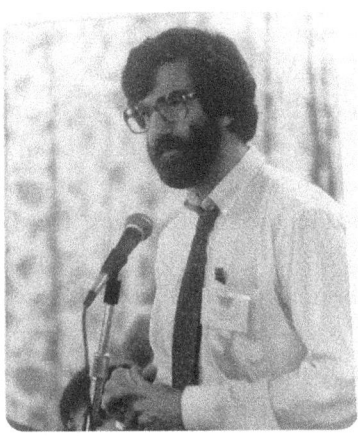

"It's like déjà vu all over again."

—Yogi Berra

Teaching accounts for much of psychology's life and influence, and so, too, for me and my career. As we've established on the first floor, most likely you have had a class of some sort in psychology. But if not, you lucky souls, even better. But some of you have gone on to multiple psych classes, or a degree in it, and, like me (heaven forbid!), a career in psychology of some kind. If so, redemption is both possible and near for us both.

My learning to be a teacher began eventfully in my graduate student days in the master's program in experimental psychology. Do I have to tell you it didn't go so well? I will: It didn't. There were three primary incidents, or episodes, (and a "bonus" fourth) that nearly drove me out of psychology and teaching forever (and probably should have, according to some of my students and certain administrators).

The first horror began during my teaching assistantship under a professor in an intro psych course. About halfway through the course, the professor, who I think never really liked me, told me I needed to take one of his classes and teach it instead of him. Unfortunately, he attended it and watched me intently. I don't remember the topic—it might have been abnormal psychology—what later became my favorite course to teach as a professor. This was different, and an inauspicious beginning. My first real lecture.

The class was a big one, about 200 students in a large amphitheater rising above me on the stage. I was nervous. No, I was petrified. Somehow, I got through it. Retreating to the professor's side at the end, he decided to give me feedback. "Do you know how many times you said 'okay'? *356!*" You can imagine the look of devastation on my face when he told me. He'd spent the whole time counting how many times I said "okay." What an Adam Henry, I thought angrily (ask a police officer what this means. I refuse to say it), though mostly I was humiliated. Time to leave psychology. It was not the career for me.

My second exercise in deciding I would never teach again was worse. As graduate teaching assistants, we were required to sometimes sit in for professors who could not come in to teach. This professor was a practicing alcoholic, near retirement, who would come into class drunk, put her head down on the desk in front of the class, press the play button on an old reel-to-reel tape recorder in front of her, and the lecture would commence. When she was sent to rehab and then fired, I learned we TAs had to take over her class in child psychology. Needless to say, I knew nothing about it. My name came up and I was scheduled for a lecture, which would determine who would take over the course. I was terrified.

Appreciating that I didn't know much about the subject, the biology and psychology of early child development, I had the foresight to ask Kerry, former fraternity brother of mine and a bio major, to come in case I needed help answering questions. I showed up for the class, nonsensically scribbled notes in hand, and stood before my professor who was sitting in the front row—glaringly.

Have you ever had your mind go blank? Mine did. I had a meltdown and couldn't even get the first word out: brain off-line, dark space. I froze, blood rushing from my head, seeing black, trying not to faint. I must have somehow indicated my panic to my buddy, also in the front row, and he got up and gave the lecture, I think from my silent plea for "help." My professor stomped out and slammed the door. Devastation. I remember I went home and cried. I decided that night I was never going to teach, I would never become a psychologist, and I would withdraw from the program right away.

My third and fourth teaching trials were not quite as eventful, though they were still embarrassing enough to sentence me to any other career but teaching and by proxy, psychology. There was the Intro Psych discussion lab that ran a betting pool on how long it would take me to kick over my full coffee cup, which was resting on the floor in front of me. I thought the cheering from the students was merely for my particularly great teaching points or jokes—but come to find out it was by the ones who won the pool as I kicked over the cup. I only learned of this later when dating the prettiest girl in the class, who confided in me.

A fourth episode of teaching idiocy occurred when I taught nearly a full two hours with my fly open in front of the class of about 40 students. I thought they were just giggling at my stupid attempts at humor, until, that is, when a helpful male compatriot in the front row held up a makeshift sign: "XYZ." Thanks. Embarrassed, I don't remember if I turned around to take care of the issue or did it right in front of everyone. But I walked out of that outright-laughing class and did not return.

From Taught to Teaching Professor
Fast forward a few years. It's now the late 1980s and '90s and I not only became an experienced teaching professor, but was promoted to full professor, despite all the good reasons I should not have been (I'm joking, sort of). I've probably taught or attempted to teach more than 10,000 of you over my 40-year academic career. Chances are that one of my former students is reading this book right now. To all:

thank you and please accept my sincerest apologies. What a blessing and honor it was to serve, attempt to teach, and drive you crazy—my outlandishness notwithstanding.

We professors can be taskmasters with a smile, a stick, and a carrot, as the saying goes (sans smile). I guess our goal was to try to prepare—or at least warn—young students about the need to be responsible and goal-directed in their pursuit of a possible career in psychology, or at least in life more generally. The following is a couple of examples of this sincere but sometimes dubious attempt to be that kind of teacher and role model.

I had just completed my first day in my course on health psychology—my specialty field—and as typical at the end of the class, there was a small group of new students waiting to talk with, and sometimes at, me. I got to them one at a time, with my research and teaching assistants nearby, answering their questions, until one student remained. "Professor Martin," she said in a tone of irritation and not a little condescension, "your syllabus and assignments, including that huge paper, treat us as if *you* were the only class we had. That is too much work for one course!" As I stared at this unknowingly stupid freshman or sophomore, with her uppity tone, my research assistants let out inaudible gasps as they anticipated their professor's response—whom they knew didn't suffer this kind of insolence lightly.

But the blast didn't come. A different sort of "wisdom" overcame my irritation and I told her, slowly, with a smile: "Welcome to the University." I think she dropped the class. Good. (Success!) I didn't do well with spoiled whiners and complainers—unless of course, it was me. Not that it ever would or could be!

Nevertheless, I was blessed with many wonderful students whom I more truly welcomed to the university and remember fondly, from my many research and teaching assistants over the years to those very special ones with whom I played a more important role as a mentor. Some of those memorable ones were just students who took one course from me.

I remember one student in particular. He was a terrible student, but a young man I liked a lot. I remember him because he walked up to me unsteadily at the beginning of the first exam, handed it back to me blank, and confessed—reeking of alcohol—that he didn't think he was in any condition to take it. I agreed, and he left. I liked that honesty.

He was not done with me, nor I with him apparently. He failed the class that semester, and then reappeared for something called "grade replacement" a year later. He asked if I remembered him, and of course, I did. He failed his second try at the class and I didn't see him again for some years. It might have been five years later when he reappeared once again. I think he was a little surprised that I remembered him so well (and fondly, as it happened). He wanted my permission to take my class a third time, as it was the last class he needed for his degree.

So, I asked him about his life and what he had been doing. He explained with this joyful light in his eyes that he had gone out and gotten this great job (because he had to), was making good money, traveling a lot, and moving up in the company. But he had been advised by other (might I say "idiot") professors and so-called friends, that he should quit that dream job and go back to finish the degree he started. WHAT? I told him that he would be *crazy* to do that. He was doing what we in the university were there to help students find and achieve. He was there! I think I might have threatened to slap him (but that would be student abuse, right?) if he even considered quitting that job to take my course and get his stupid degree. I might not have said "stupid" degree, but that's what I thought. I think he was about to kiss me; he was so thrilled with my advice. He didn't quit his job and enroll in my class. I would not have let him!

Off to the Medical School Setting!
My teaching travails high-hurdled, or detoured, from the university classroom to the medical school setting. My appointment to the medical school where I was also a VA staff psychologist brought other unique teaching experiences that I remember well. One of my department of psychiatry and human-behavior roles was to teach the clinical interview to the medical students. My first, pitiful try was a post-lunch hour lecture for the third-year medical students, M3s. I

was great at putting most of the students to sleep halfway through the lecture. I later learned that it wasn't just my terribly boring, hypnotic teaching style, but that most of those med students had been up all night covering the various hospital wards and the ER, and had just eaten lunch. Result: sleep.

The medical school was no stranger to teacher "fun." I recall hearing about a hilarious (not to the affected med students, of course) "hazing" of M3s (poor folks). It goes with the territory and part of the humility-based learning curve. When participating in their first rounds with the medical staff, they were singled out to conduct a quick diabetes test on a patient by sticking a finger in the patient's urine-filled bedpan and tasting it for sugar spilling. It would have been a sweet taste if in diabetics, I'm told, but what do I know, I never tried it. Each M3 had to, one by one, stick a finger in and taste, just like the attending or resident physician did before them. What they didn't notice is that the finger the staff used was not the same finger they tasted—unlike the unsuspecting M3s, who all used the same finger. Ugh. But what fun. By the way, urine is supposedly sterile, so no problem.

But we also taught small groups of med students, and for one class I was a star. No, not because my teaching and training were so outstanding, but because I threw out a student who walked in late, halfway through the semester. I didn't recognize him, so as he was looking for an empty desk, I confronted him: "Who are you?" He declared in his med student privilege voice, "I'm _____. I'm in your class." To his (and the class's) great surprise, I actually threw him out. I'd had it with a student who would think he could get away with this kind of behavior, and decided an important lesson was in order for him and possibly for the whole class. It worked for one (the class, I believe) and hopefully for the student. When he finally agreed to leave, I turned back to the class to apologize for my being so harsh with the student and for the class disruption. But they gave me applause! (It might have been standing room kind.) I was told that he had done that in all of his medical school classes, and I was the *first* professor who had refused to put up with it and thrown him out!

I was nominated for "best professor" in the medical school later that year. I was convinced it was only from that incident (not from my spectacular teaching) that the nomination came. I did not win. Darn.

Simplifiers and Complicators
Learning how to teach had as much to do with learning how *not* to do it, of which I had quite a bit of experience. I had a colleague and close friend (RK) from my university department who had written a statistics textbook that was a marvel of understandability. He told me something I've always remembered. There are two kinds of people: complicators and simplifiers.

I figure to be a simplifier you need to have a mastery of the subject, like a clown diver needs to be an expert at all the dives before screwing around, making it funny, and not dying. My buddy and colleague was a simplifier who could make the most complicated subject understandable. Like statistics. My stat teacher was a complicator, who could take an already complicated subject and overcomplicate it further! I think he, my friend and colleague, was the one who taught me about that difference in teaching and learning.

More Teaching Mishaps
So I determined to become a simplifier and not a complicator in all aspects of my professional life—including (stupidly it turned out) in teaching. But in my ramp-up to becoming a simplifier in all areas of practice, I decided to try: *Simplify Statistics for Right-Brained Therapists by Not Ever Using Numbers or Formulas.* SAY WHAT? You heard me.

I tried it in one of my teaching (summer break) jobs at a local independent graduate school for training therapists. What an opportunity! I thought it was going well. I was teaching probability, t- and F-tests, analysis of variance (ANOVA), and how you would use them to determine differences between experimental groups—all without numbers or formulas. This was my first big mistake. Then I gave them an essay-based statistics exam (second big mistake) in which they picked their own research question (third big mistake), created the design and chose the method of analysis (fourth big mistake), made up the data, and interpreted the results. To top it off, I gave them unlimited time to complete what was supposed to be a two-hour final exam. When some students were still working on it (tears and blood streaking down onto their papers) SIX HOURS LATER, I finally had to get them to finish so I could make the long drive up the mountains to my home. Phew.

What I read in their exams was not so much a reflection of their senseless knowledge and understanding of experimental design and statistics (little to none), but of my truly ridiculous teaching idea and approach. My student evaluations were quite pointed and not very nice to their loving professor/would-be simplifier. Would you believe I was accused of forcing them to take a six-hour final exam? I was. The other comments were not so uplifting. I never taught that course again at that school.

I recall another humiliating teaching experience worth mentioning in the "how not to do it" school. This lesson was large and extra mortifying. I was a research professor giving a lecture at the National Institutes of Health (NIH) before distinguished colleagues based on my NIH-funded research on exercise and high blood pressure. You might remember or have heard about the old carousel slide projectors. Well, at some point in the lecture, probably very early, one of my damnable cardboard backing slides jammed. Several of us descended on the slide projector. One of the highly unhelpful helpers pulled the carousel off the projector, while another unhelpful colleague undid the locking piece, and a third (you're getting the idea) turned the slide carousel over in a heroic effort to find and unjam the bent and crushed slide. This combination of "helpfulness" resulted in all of my fifty-or-so slides falling onto the floor in no particular order.

I spent the next 15 minutes (it felt like 15 hours) picking up individual slides, peering at them in the light, and trying to order them so I could conduct my lecture with the audience staring at me in silence the whole time. Horrifyingly embarrassing! I heard a week or two later from a well-known colleague with whom I was collaborating on a book. He asked me how it went at NIH with the slideshow!

Ouch! He heard about the slideshow from across the country. I was finished! But, sadly, to students of the future, I wasn't—with the fortunate exception of abnormal psychology.

Abnormal Psych by the Abnormal Psychologist
Nevertheless, in some classes I did a pretty good job teaching. Abnormal psych became one of my favorite courses to teach ever, being so abnormal myself. I couldn't help wondering if it helps (or is necessary) to have the same disorder or disorders you are working with or teaching. Another "good question," I'm guessing.

But my best version of my course on Abnormal Psychology was the semester I decided to recruit guest speakers who had those disorders, sans, of course, me. (I wasn't ready then or prepared for full disclosure such as in this book.) When I put out the call for people, the students knew, who might be willing to come in and talk about their mental illness, I was surprised at how many volunteers I got. My church also had lots of the "mentally ill" (including me, of course), who had recovered, been healed, or gotten good treatment, and whose lives were stable again.

In fact, my favorite and the class's favorite from church was a guy who was a classic psychopath/sociopath who had been in prison for murdering two people—both of whom he said deserved it. He found God in prison and his lifetime sentence was reduced due to good behavior. When he described to the class what it was like to kill someone (he was in the Mexican Mafia), every eye was glued on him and his story. He represented the classic sociopath disorder, and his sharing powerfully reflected that fact. The most frightening part was when he answered the question from the class whether he felt remorse for those murders. He stated, without apparent emotion, that he did not.

Other "abnormal" guests had a variety of conditions, including one girl with multiple personality disorder (now called dissociative identity disorder or DID). The students were hoping to get to see one of her "alters" or different personalities that she described but didn't transition into (darn). There was also a 19-year-old new army draftee who, while deployed in Saigon, Vietnam at the height of the war, was assigned the job of putting the body parts of American soldiers and Marines into body bags and coffins. His was one of the worst cases of PTSD I have ever seen. I think my unique and successful approach to this course helped me think more strategically about how best to teach and motivate my students.

Motivational Teaching

Somewhat later in my teaching career, when I was becoming an expert in the area of motivation science and counseling[3], I couldn't help but wonder—would it be possible to apply these motivational techniques to my psychology courses? It made sense. Here's how it went:

I would give a reading assignment for the following class, and during that class I would *not lecture* the students. Rather, I would start the class by asking them what they thought of the readings. As you might imagine, I got lots of blank stares and silence. Sometimes I would probe and mention a topic or two that was in the unit or materials, but other times not. Strategically, I designed the class to have a quiz at the end of each weekly class. The quizzes were worth roughly 50 percent of the total course grade—so it was a fearful thing when I announced over their stupefied silence to my questions, "Great, then since there are no questions, you must all be ready for our quiz."

At that point—surprise!—hands were thrust up in the air, books and articles were cracked open, and the rustle of page-turning broke the dumb, silent fog over the classroom. So we were underway. I didn't answer their questions but wrote them on the board. Summarizing their questions, I asked what others could tell us about that topic, what the book and reading materials had to say, and whether they understood, bought it, etc. This led to a lively, collaborative dialogue between students and their teacher, even some interesting personal stories related to the issues. I then, after picking their coming-to-life brains, asked if they would like to know what I thought about those questions and areas—yes they did! And I proceeded to share some of my thoughts and a few examples, being careful not to fully answer. I might have suggested other literature for them to check, for example over the internet, to find their own answers.

Then we together would organize the questions and issues into the order they thought best, followed by a summary (filling the whiteboard) of what they told me the book and literature said, along with their own opinions. When we agreed they were ready for the quiz, we did it. This same process was repeated each new class period, for the whole course. But I stopped shortly thereafter, only using it for probably one more course. Not every course fit into the daily or weekly quiz mode, and bottom line, students wanted, and sometimes needed, to be spoon-fed information that only I was the expert over. Looking back, transforming all my courses into this motivational approach would have been a great sabbatical year focus. But I had the sabbatical travel bug and never got around to it.

Teaching Revenge
Sometimes my students could be rough on a young professor learning to teach, particularly about those courses not in his specialty area. But I got back at those degenerate students and mockers one time, with a different kind of fun motivation—mine. The payback was sweet as honey.

You see, I had a full beard for years and then one day I decided in a wild hair notion to shave it all off. Crazy. I looked *so* different my dog didn't even recognize me. From there, my evil student–abusing mind got an idea: I could go into class wearing different kinds of clothes and carrying a strange-looking briefcase that I never used, and tell them I was my brother, David! So I did. I said, "Dr. Martin was called away and he asked me as his brother to take the class for the day." I told them that I (David) knew absolutely *nothing* about psychology but that I could tell stories about my brother, John, if they would like to hear them." "YES!" the class enthusiastically responded, and we were off to the humiliating (of John) races!

I don't remember what stories I told, but they were crazy and fun, and all made me look like a nut. (Of course, I weaved enough psychology into the stories to cover myself should I be criticized for not teaching psychology.) And what a lively class it was. It was so interesting to watch the students' faces during the class, some with that quizzical look of disbelief—was I really my brother, and was any of this true?—but most seemed to buy the story.

The next class when I returned, transitioned back to Professor Martin with normal clothes, hairstyle (still sans beard) and bookbag, I confessed the hilarious deception, though not all thought it was so stunt-worthy. Hey, please don't tell my university. I am emeritus there and I might have that rescinded. Really. But to readers who were students in that class, you will remember me and that day. I hope you were one of those with the good sense of ridiculous humor, and not one of those humorless bad students. If the latter, don't bother contacting me. I will pretend not to have received or read your nasty confrontation. The statute of limitations on student abuse has passed.

Mentors and Mentees: Supervisory Teaching Fun
My roles as a teacher, clinical supervisor, and mentor oftentimes blended to become one and the same, and I was mentored in these areas by (as I've said) one of the best. It was indeed hard supervising myself, much less others, but I was a willing subject either way. My own major professor, doctoral thesis advisor, and mentor taught me to be a teacher, researcher, writer, supervisee, and then supervisor and mentor. This all happened through his role modeling and forceful efforts to mold me, and for the most part it worked. After all, I did become a teacher, professor, clinical supervisor, psychologist, and research mentor. (But a writer? The jury is still out on that one.)

Some of my attempts at creative but useful "fun" with students overflowed to other arenas including my clinical supervision. I was a clinical practicum supervisor for much of my career as a mentor for training master's and especially doctoral students in clinical psychology. I learned by being mentored by some of the best. I passed on quite a lot to my mentees along the training way, including behavior modification strategies, trauma and PTSD interventions, motivational science approaches to counseling, addictions treatment and communication, and finally, faith and spiritually oriented integration with evidence-based cognitive behavioral and faith-based motivational interventions.

When I was a clinical supervisor for doctoral students learning to be therapists, I remembered some occasions when I could build fires under them in enjoyably effective ways. Sometimes those clinical fires had as much smoke as flame, but one in particular was pure flame.

One student trainee had just come from attempting to counsel a client in our university psychology clinic. As usual, he came with videotape in hand (and in this case, tail between his legs) for us to go over the embarrassment of a session. And it was. It only took a minute or two of watching to discover the client was drunk. I could practically smell the alcohol through the video! Instead of kindly stopping the tape and discussing with the student about not ever trying to counsel a client who is drunk or high (since you would be "counseling" the drug and not the person, besides the fact they would remember little or none about the session), I decided to make the student suffer through the whole hour tape, without word from me. It was powerful lesson time. Then, at the end, after a good deal of embarrassment and seat-squirming by him, we had our discussion about counseling a drunk or drug addict. It was painful for the student, purposely on my part, for that wonderful "one trial learning" opportunity. He likely never tried that again.

But I wasn't done with him. There was another important learning opportunity I didn't want to let pass. I asked how did the client get to the clinic? He drove was the answer. Hmmm. I asked whether he offered to call the client a cab (Uber hadn't been invented then) or a family member to come get him. "Yes," he responded, "but he wanted to drive himself and refused." "Did you ask for his car keys?" "No. I couldn't do that. It would have been bad for our rapport." Say what? Given that he was about to use a lethal weapon (car) while dangerously toxic with alcohol, I asked calmly, did he consider calling the police to come pick him up and save him or another from being killed? (MADD also was not around then.) "No, that would have been unethical." I ended up assuring him that even if the client had tried to sue him for this "breach" of ethics, and possible illegal violation of his confidentiality and privacy rights, that no jury or judge would ever find him, the therapist, guilty of anything other than following higher ethics, protecting the client, himself, and other unsuspecting drivers. Lesson two? Maybe.

I remember another creative supervisory adventure. My very good female student (this was Heidi; I talk about her later in the veterans PTSD chapter) was referred a woman who was fairly seriously depressed with suicidal thoughts. She had been prescribed antidepressant medication but was in crisis during the few weeks while the medication was rising to effective blood levels in her brain. So we added an intervention during the counseling that could help her during that transition—physical exercise *during* counseling!

Both the student trainee and the client were regular exercisers, and fit, though the client had not been exercising much lately. We know that especially aerobic exercise such as brisk walking, running, swimming, or biking can produce similar brain chemistry changes as stimulated by the most effective antidepressant medications—serotonin and dopamine increases in the neurotransmitters. The client liked the idea, so dual verbal and physical "counseling" it was!

The sessions commenced with brisk walks around the clinic facility. In addition, we instituted a DRO intervention, or differential reinforcement of other behavior. Whenever the client began to talk about all the reasons she was depressed and her life was terrible (which we had already determined and discussed but would only further depress her), the counselor trainee would turn her head away from the client, pick up the pace, and not respond verbally to her. When the opposite happened or was prompted by the counselor—positive or neutral talk—the counselor slowed the pace, turned, smiled, and looked at and talked with the client. Brilliant, right? Maybe. I do think it worked well enough to help the client during this critical period awaiting the extra boost in mood from the medication, and also began the all-important and strategic CBT (the most evidence-supported psychological approach to depression) to help her manage and modify her depressive thoughts and behavior.

CAN WE TALK?

Healthy Depression and Anxiety. Is there such a thing? Yep. Now maybe we are using different definitions here, and this is a place where you therapists, psychologists, psychiatrists, and your clients—not to mention the fields of clinical psychology and psychiatry as a whole—will strongly differ with me. But bear with me here.

There is the *dis-ease* of depression and anxiety on the one hand, and the diseases or formal depression and anxiety *disorders* on the other. They are different but can overlap quite significantly. For example, there are many circumstances in life that can cause a "normal" depression or anxiety state—it's the body and mind telling us there is something wrong in our lives that needs attention and hopefully healing or fixing. We have sometimes termed this "reactive depression"—as opposed to biologic or organic depression. Consider the loss of a loved one through death or divorce, job loss, relationship breakup, or children troubles. There are many situations that cause us to feel depressed or to grieve. That is normal, human reaction. Sometimes I will affirm the person in their situation by saying something like: "No wonder you are depressed (or anxious), given what has happened. Let's see what might be best to help you get through this period." These may be times, for instance grieving over the loss of a family member, where the best therapy is the love and care of a friend who is good at listening, affirming, and not directing or "fixing" you. There are many around us, as well as social fellowships like 12-Step and church programs, that facilitate a more natural processing and healing such that professional help, including medication, may not always be needed or helpful. I hope you have those kinds of people in your life. If not, go find and hang on to them.

In our tobacco treatment project working with smokers from the AA program, we discovered a strange type of depression—one that surfaced paradoxically when they quit or cut down significantly on their cigarette use. It didn't make sense until we understood it as a conditioned effect of "parting the smoke screen" that blocked old emotional wounds and memories dating back to when they first began smoking and using mood-altering drugs. This phenomenon led us to include cognitive therapy for depression for our smoking clients, especially as an additional treatment for smoking relapse prevention.

But it's when depression or anxiety is present for an extended time and has a more generalized negative effect on multiple sides of the person's life that therapy and medication can be needed or most helpful. Be careful though, as you may not need therapy or medication, and just by seeing professionals who do that as their business could push you into a longer-term (or lifetime) path of those things that may not be necessary—at least for that length of time—to say nothing of how expensive it can be!

Medications for psychological problems have typically only been investigated and demonstrated effectiveness for shorter term use, such as six or nine months. That is not to say that you do not need to continue with a regimen after that, but it may be that you do not. How will you know if you never experience a drug holiday like the kind that the psychiatry department at a medical school I was on the faculty of used to do with all their psychotropic medication–prescribed patients. They would fade medications down under careful supervision to see whether or how much medication was then needed or useful. This should not be done on your own but under careful medical and psychological monitoring.

Now I guess you can say—THAT'S IT. NOW YOU HAVE RUINED PSYCHOLOGY AND PSYCHIATRY FOR ME! Or this is when you want to burn this book and file suit against me. But you can't. Remember our informed consent and my liability protection.

Suggestion: Determine whether your depression or anxiety is of a normal reactive type, which will likely be helped when your circumstances or the external causes change (such as grieving over loss), gradually heal, or stimulate you to change something in your life that is the cause of it. Loving friends or family can help with

> this wisdom, so seek them out. Get professional help if the depression or anxiety condition runs deeper and affects your life in some more significant and enduring ways. These are very common conditions and there are many effective treatments that can help—particularly the evidence-supported CBT and medications. But find a person or people to talk about it no matter what.
>
> *Suicidality.* Lastly, if you are or you know of someone struggling with thoughts of suicide (not just occasionally with no plan to act on it), talk with someone or with them about it, then seek help—first from others and then from a professional. But talk. Troubled teens, elders, and veterans with PTSD are especially vulnerable to suicidal depression. Don't be afraid to ask them about it. You will not give them the idea—they already have it. Loving listening can go a long way toward helping them back to life, and don't delay in connecting with them and keeping the connection. If you think they are seriously suicidal (maybe with a specific plan and means to kill themselves), DO NOT LEAVE THEM ALONE. Either you, a family member, or a friend should be with them until professional help and/or the suicidal depression passes or lessens significantly. Finally, consider getting trained in suicide prevention through a program like ASIST or others. It can save a life—sort of like CPR for depression and suicidality. What would happen if half of our population got this training, similarly to the public health goal for getting 50 percent of everyone trained in CPR for heart attacks? Think about it.

Cognitive and behavioral therapies are joined by motivational approaches[4] in helping people to change and heal. In one memorable example, a client in the training clinic was a very successful 30ish professional woman who was painfully shy, not so attractive, and wanted to find a man to marry and with whom to have a family. We used a motivational strategy, asking for her top life values (getting married and having a family was number one) and comparing them to her lifestyle and behaviors (seeking time or dates with eligible men was not even on her behavioral radar much less repertoire).

So, we became Columbo-like (you might remember the series with Peter Falk as the typically confused investigator who would get criminals to help him put them in jail by playing "dumb"), using confusion and gently provocative (and paradoxical) arguing against her top goal. The therapist pretended to be confused and dumb, suggesting that the discrepancy between her value and behavior indicated she might need to change the value and move it way down her list.

This provocative "reframe" elicited a (hoped for) passionate objection from the client, who decided to change her behavior to be more consistent with her top value—marriage and family—which she had refused to change. With this new motivation springing up and shifting in the client, a creative brainstorming collaboration between her therapist and her resulted in the enlistment of an attractive doctoral student to role-play with her and teach her to flirt and approach suitable men. The videos and feedback did the trick. Next thing we knew she was dressing more attractively, joining clubs with single men and women, and even asking men out on dates. As I write this, I'm certain she is married with kids while continuing her professional success as well. If she is reading this, congratulations. Send me pictures of you and your family!

CAN WE TALK?

Motivating the Unmotivated. There is a style of talking with people that comes from the science of motivational communication. It's usually called motivational interviewing[3-5].

Motivational Style of Talking to Others:

1. *Know the Law of Reciprocity.* It's like a judo match. For every action or force against a person, an equal and opposite reaction will occur. If you want them to come in your direction (physically or mindfully), the worst thing you can do is to pull, push, or drag them. They will react—normally—to this pressure, and resist. Sometimes gently pushing them away can cause a shift towards you or what you think is a better way to think about something. (For

example: "Maybe you are right. This is something too hard for you. It probably will never happen."). But be careful. This can backfire!

2. *Reflective Listening.* Listen, don't tell, correct, or judge. They don't work and will only raise resistance to change.

3. *Advice. Don't give unsolicited or unwanted advice.* A Chinese proverb says: Advice—wise people don't need it; fools won't heed it. Better to ask the person what he or she thinks best. But, when you think the person is ready to receive some helpful advice, *ask permission to give advice.*

4. *Affirmations.* Praise and affirmations work well and can be greatly encouraging to a person's motivation. Don't skimp on this.

5. *Autonomy.* Support the person's freedom to choose or change, with a comment like, "Only you can decide whether to do this or to change. What do you think you would like or need to do?"

6. *Collaborate, Don't Manage.* Walk with the person as a collaborator, not as a manager or director. Sometimes we can help a person get "unstuck" in an area of their life—when they are ready and perhaps ask for help.

7. *Ready, Willing, Able.* People change when they are ready, willing, and able to change. There is timing and patience involved. Pushing and pulling verbally doesn't work (unless you are in the military or prison, and if so, ignore all this). We can help people get ready, decide, and be willing, and even to have the skills to do something—but only as they see us as a caring, gentle guide (at most), partner, or collaborator.

Belonephobia

I expressed more of my creative supervisory brilliance at the VA as a staff psychologist working with one of the many excellent psychology resident/interns under me. I once got a referral from the cancer service of the hospital for a patient with brain cancer, whose tumor had apparently returned. However, they were not able to conduct testing that required injection of dye for imaging. He had just *knocked out cold* the phlebotomist who came at him with the needle. He had a needle phobia—called belonephobia of all things. Turns out he had a traumatic reaction to the experience of being repeatedly punctured with catheter needles during a previous procedure in which he had collapsed veins and they could not get a good line in. So, *nobody* was going to get anywhere near him with a needle. Hence, the referral to psychology and right in my target zone as head of the behavioral medicine program.

So with an intern working under me, we conducted standard imaginal desensitization of the feared needles, but the patient became too panicked at even the word, imagined picture, or thoughts of going through injections with needles. He was unable to become or maintain deep relaxation necessary for that therapy. Next step was to consider a chemical "assist" by having him receive oral (not IV—get it?) sedation. But he refused that because he did not want anything mood altering/drugging him, as he was a recovering drug addict and wanted to remain free of that drugged feeling and violation of his abstinence. Hmmm. What to do. We were kind of stuck. Then I had an idea.

What about exercising him to exhaustion? As a runner and sometime marathoner, I knew what it felt like to be physically exhausted and unable to be mentally aroused at anything. You are just like a person looks (and feels) when they are deeply relaxed—a limp rag. I knew that a person cannot really continue to be highly anxious, mentally, when their body and muscles are deeply relaxed in a state of physical exhaustion. We talked with the patient and his family, and arranged with the cardiology department to provide a medical resident and a treadmill for this purpose. All agreed, including the patient's deeply religious Christian family, who were enlisted to pray in the hospital chapel during the procedure—and all went well.

The patient, who was cleared to exercise intensely, was put on a treadmill and run through a medically supervised, graded-exercise test protocol which, with its rapid progressive elevations, would wear our patient out quickly and bring him to exhaustion. For the procedure,

I was stationed at a table in another part of the room, complete with blood pressure cuff and manual inflator, and the phlebotomist (hiding needle with dye) dressed in street clothes (no provocative, scary surgical garb). After the exercise protocol was completed, the exhausted patient was led to the table where I stood between him and the phlebotomist (with hidden syringe), placed the BP cuff on him, and began pumping it up. Then the phlebotomist walked up behind me and injected the patient, who was too tired and distracted to react. Success. The family's prayers worked too. And no one was knocked out either (especially not me or the needle-wielding phlebotomist).

I kept encouraging the intern under me to write it up as a clinical report for a psychology journal. But she never did. Neither did I. It was on to another clinical program, student intern supervision, or research study. Could have gotten a nice publication too.

THIRD FLOOR

PSYCHOLOGICAL ADVENTURES AND MISADVENTURES

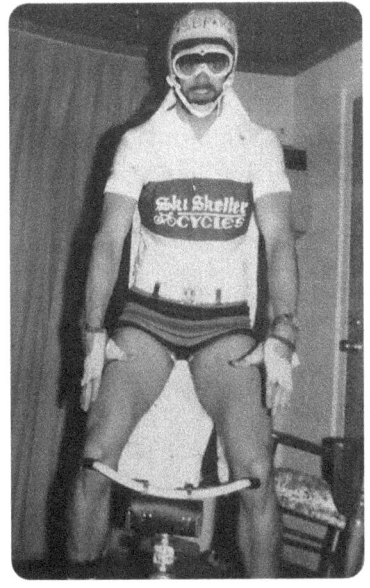

Picture taken just prior to your author's winning tricycle race at a local bar near the children's hospital where he worked as a special ed teacher, irony noted.

"Great moments in science: Einstein discovers that time is actually money."

—GARY LARSON

"Show me a sane man [excluding your author—see above pic] and I will cure him for you."

—DR. CARL G. JUNG

The third floor is a psychological depository of random adventures and misadventures reflecting the abnormal life of a psychologist and would-be scientist, student trainee, and psychiatry "fun." Included are chapters on my earlier clinical consultation in the VA hospital, some fun with clinical training and research craziness, and travels around the world to export my professor nuttiness via that brilliant invention of the seven-year sabbatical. This is all capped with some random professional junk food (having nothing at all to do with food) misadventures that I couldn't find any other place to put. I trust you will have some enjoyment if not good fun with these crazy stories, confessions, and revelations. Unfortunately, there might even be some learning involved, but that was accidental and unintended for this section. Please forgive me.

ROOM 301

CLINICAL CONSULTATION PSYCHOLOGY

"The way most of us seek to help others is more like wrestling than dancing."

—Marcus Aurelius (121–180)

The Consultation Service

I learned a tremendous amount from my time as a new consulting psychologist working in the veterans administration hospital—mistakes and all (fortunately nobody died, so far as I knew, that is).

A primary role for me at the VA, my first psychologist position, was to run the behavioral medicine consultation service. Physicians throughout the VA hospital who needed or wanted some assistance from the psychology service could send a written consult to us. Then I would either go myself or have a psych intern under me answer the consult question in writing with a formal typed report. Their consult might only say something like "evaluate," giving us (frustratingly) no further information on why or for what. When we got enough of an idea by looking at the patient's chart, a lengthy evaluation report would follow a few days later. It's the way I was trained to conduct an evaluation. Was I ever wrong.

I managed to make a sufficient number of medical staff upset at us, and me in particular, in my first learning year by this ignorant practice. Oftentimes the patient would have been discharged by then, without help from psychology! But our consultation report was a thing of beauty, though never read (just fumed over). So I learned to find the one who made the consult and talk with him or her directly. "What do you need, and how can we help?" For example, they just wanted to know if the patient was crazy, whether the complaints were psychological and not medical, or whether they were faked (malingering). But the consulting doctor couldn't write that on the consult. And they needed the report placed in the patient's chart within 24 hours to state the consult was received and being acted upon. I later learned to talk to the nurses on the ward the patient was on, especially the head nurse. It didn't take long for me to learn who runs the hospital and the wards: the nurses! A *very* valuable lesson!

Chronic Pain Clinic
I can't recall whether I inherited this clinic or I created it. Heaven help me if I created it. But the need was there, especially for our many injured, wounded, and disabled vets. The inpatients referred to me would often come with a shopping cart full of old charts in tow. This was not a good sign. When I heard those shopping-cart wheels squeak, wobbling on the floor coming psychology's way, I knew it was for me. Get ready.

I soon learned how to counsel these usually angry, hurting, and frustrated, pain patients and never to get in a discussion with them about whether it was psychological or physical pain. They wanted to talk about that since their physicians had essentially accused them of only having the pain in their heads—especially ironic if headaches were part of their medical symptoms. I would explain that a good part of all pain was the suffering that came from the psychological side and not only the organic cause. I learned to always affirm their physical pain and told them I couldn't help with that, but I probably could with the other side of the pain that came from suffering, stress, and life breakdown. At some point, we could begin to look at what was possible in improving their whole-life adaptation while trying to minimize the pain and suffering.

We were receiving enough pain patient referrals to consider starting an outpatient chronic pain program. So I did. One of their homework assignments was to keep a record of their (three-times-a-day) pain ratings, relaxation practice times, and physical exercise.

But many of these wily vets knew the system and how to work it to avoid seemingly dumb and cumbersome prescriptions by me, the head shrinker. According to them, they were not crazy, they just needed better medications and hopefully a medical cure! Not surprisingly, most were dependent on highly addictive pain meds, and part of our program included collaborating with the medical staff to reduce the dose or wean them off those medications—another role for which the vets so loved us.

Anyway, after looking at a number of their self-monitoring forms, I eventually found a strange similarity in most of them: they looked the same—same pen, often same data each day and week, and unwrinkled iron-flat paper forms—unlike what you would expect if they had been carrying them around in their pockets day-to-day. When I caught them filling out the weekly forms in the waiting room for the upcoming session, that gave me an idea about what was up.

Exercise and relaxation homework was no different. We suspected the exercise data may have been corrupted in a similar, nefarious way. The pedometers we had issued them to wear every day to track walking and movement were found to have a higher number of steps than expected—we caught them shaking them by hand in that same waiting room before we showed up for the session! Then there were the relaxation practice tapes. That was an easy "fake"—the vets often would just record on their forms that they had done it. Simple. But for once, I outsmarted these bright deceiving patients by recording a special code or "hidden word" on some of the tapes (we gave them different cassette tapes for each prescribed relaxation) but not all. They had to note which ones had the special embedded code or word and which didn't. The "hidden marker" technique—a great idea, I thought! Nevertheless, they found the best way to circumvent this and other "checkups" on them—they just wouldn't show up for the outpatient group! Oh well.

Hypertension Clinic
A big problem in the treatment of hypertension or high blood pressure was medication compliance, and I received many consults to

help with noncompliance or nonadherence to these VA patients' often lifesaving medication regimens. We were asking our vets who had high blood pressure to take a pill that made them feel bad, for something that didn't make them feel bad. See the problem? No wonder their medication compliance was not so good. In fact, hypertension is called the "silent killer" because it *doesn't* have symptoms, that is, until the later stages or during acute episodes that might include stroke or heart attack.

We tried having them record their medication taking, but soon learned, similarly to the chronic pain clinic, not to trust their self-reports. It was just too tempting to not tell the whole truth. Even pill counts were not so accurate (it was too easy to dump some extra pills that they failed to take). We got permission from the hospital to add to their antihypertensive prescription a "tracer," vitamin B2, which fluoresces the urine. It wouldn't hurt them and could improve their vitamin intake. We would then ask for urine samples, and one of my research assistants—who was our "pee gal"—would check their urine under the florescent lamp. Fun job. She had a great sense of humor fortunately, and went on, incidentally, to enter medical school (probably to get away from this pee project)!

My work in the area of heart disease, and specifically hypertension, led me to investigate the effect exercise had on high blood pressure (a strongly positive one), and the related issue of how in the world to get these patients to develop the exercise habit. I will address this in upcoming chapters on community interventions and research.

Dialysis Ward
One of my earliest consulting experiences at the VA was with the dialysis ward. There were many vets who had kidney disease—high blood pressure damaging the kidneys—and three or four times a week for four or five hours, depending on the amount of excess fluid, they had to be filtered.

Not surprising, many of these dialysis patients were depressed—which was the reason for our being consulted. As our consults for depressed patients in the dialysis unit piled up, I decided to create an intervention program, with the unit's staff physician approval. But we did not first get, or work together with, the nurses or head nurse on that unit. Big mistake, I found.

We tried several things, and for the most part they worked well. Too well according to the nurses. WHAT? For example, we knew exercise helped their dialysis and overall health, and so we fitted patients with pedometers (we had lots left over from the chronic pain clinic that eventually had to be closed down due to nonattendance—big surprise). We measured walking at home and set up a token economy (behavior modification "speak") in which they could earn really nice walking and running shoes for walking and coming in appropriately underweight for their next dialysis session (overweight necessitated extra dialysis time, including an added day). We also paid vets with VA canteen coupons, up to 10 dollars' worth for the highest level of adherence. To earn money and receive shoe donations, I even went on the radio and TV locally, including sponsoring the VA Heart Health 5K run/walk in the community. It was all a great success, especially the improvement in the dialysis patients and their depression recovery.

But it was not a success with the nursing staff, whom I had all but ignored. Then the other shoe dropped. I was called to a special meeting with the whole staff from the unit, including the attending physician. I came with two of my interns from my behavioral medicine rotation and was told, in no uncertain terms, that psychology would no longer be needed or wanted there on the ward. When I asked why, especially given our great success story with the patients, I was told that they, the nurses, didn't think we should be paying or rewarding clients for doing the things they were *supposed* (i.e., *told*) to do.

Controlling my upset, I said: "Do you mean you still want us to leave even if the patients who were doing so well, in part from the reinforcement program we had implemented to help their depression and dialysis management, would revert to depression and noncompliance with the diet and home exercise?" Their (the head nurse's) answer: "Yes."

I was outraged. I looked over to the attending physician for support but got none. He knew, and I learned, who ran the unit. The nurses. I got up and stormed off with my interns in tow, and we were never consulted again. I blamed it all on those nurses. But after some time and further maturing experiences, I came to believe it was *my* fault, my error, for not including the nurses from the very beginning. I learned this again with the cardiology ward (you would think this would have been one-trial learning).

Cardiology Ward
My primary interest, clinically and as a researcher, was in the area of cardiovascular disease. Much of heart disease has to do with one's lifestyle choices and behaviors like lack of exercise, smoking, poor diet and stress, and poor medication adherence, so there was a lot of room for behavioral risk modification. This was my realm of psychology.

I, therefore, made it a priority to befriend the cardiologists from the heart ward, first asking and being invited as a new VA psychologist to attend weekly rounds with them and their staff. That was a good place for getting one's professional foot in the door, I found, and it worked to generate consults as I made suggestions such as: "I think we might be able to help this patient. Would you consider sending us a consult?" So the consults came, for helping with behavior change, and sometimes counseling for family who wanted to help support their husband or father in the fight against heart disease.

Another opportunity to learn who runs the ward! I think I responded to the first run of consults on cardiology patients with longer, days-delayed evaluation reports. The result was the same: irritated physicians and medical interns and residents in cardiology whose patients were discharged before we could even be of help. I think our consult found its way to the back of the patient's chart, and then was sent to the records department. Darn. As with my general consultation department, I learned pretty soon to *immediately* follow up the consultation request while contacting the referring physician *and* the nurses on the ward who knew about and had charge over that patient. This kind of important thing (d'ya think?) was not taught in graduate school, including in my clinical practicum training. Once I found out what they wanted or needed, I usually completed the consult, or at least made a longer note in their progress note, within a day. That satisfied them, temporarily at least, and gave me a little more time to complete the consult and help with the issue.

Because we were getting an increasing number of new consults from cardiology while trying to maintain contact with the discharged patients—we wanted to continue to help on an outpatient basis—I did two things. First, I created a behavioral cardiology outpatient program and clinic, and I got permission—working *very* closely with the nurses and head nurse especially this time!—to earn money and receive shoe donations to set up an inpatient program, complete with our own two-bed room. Second, we fitted patients with pedometers to measure and encourage their walking about, changed their dress code so they wore their regular clothes and not "sick role" pajamas and butt-peeking gowns.

We found, and research shows, that how a person appears and is dressed determines how they are often treated by others. This is especially true for sick people or those in a hospital setting. When they are in patient clothes, they are treated as sick people, and not expected to do much on their own, much less wander off the ward. Even the medical staff would treat these patients differently when in non-patient street clothes with "well patient" interactions and expectations.

One of the harder things for these patients, who were just post-cardiac surgery, as well as their family members, was to adhere to the doctor's recommendation to get up and walk—to earn money and receive shoe donations even the same day as the surgery. But we had a secret weapon, besides the regular clothes and pedometer tracker: Nurse Ratchet! We know there was no such thing, but we always had a nurse who would go in the patient's room and get the patient up out of bed with a command (!), especially those reluctant or unwilling to do so. They also would work with us to shoo them out of the room to walk around and put some miles on their pedometer.

Anyone who has gone on rounds or been subjected to them as a patient or bedside-standing family knows that the sicker patients get more attention. This makes sense. So, I would overtly (sometimes loudly) say: "Look at Mr. Smith there walking by in the hall, who is doing so well thanks to the nurses and the behavioral cardiology program! (I couldn't help myself.) Come in and say hi to the doctors and nurses on rounds, and show them how well you are doing."

Having learned from my wet-behind-the-ears young psychologist first year, I involved the nurses and head nurse in the behavioral cardiology program and room. We put the program together as collaborators, and nurses took ownership of it in a real way. I would always go to them for advice or consultation when there was a problem with our patients, and offer to assist with any other patients who needed help.

One time I was leading our outpatient behavioral cardiology clinic and noticed that one of our patients, who had just had a coronary bypass, did not look well. His skin was pasty white, he was sweaty and not breathing as well as he should have been. Patients who have had a bypass virtually always look much better after the blood-increasing procedure. I was concerned enough about him to approach one of my cardiology doctor friends in the hall that day and suggest he see him in their clinic, even though he was not scheduled with them for another month. He agreed to see the patient because of my strong concerns.

The next day, the cardiology doc grabbed me in the hospital hall and told me that it was good that I had him seen by them. When they hooked him up to an EKG, his heart rhythm did not look good, in fact was so abnormal that they rushed him into surgery over at the adjoining medical school. What they found was that his bypass was done on the WRONG SIDE OF HIS HEART—the right (but wrong) side. They redid the bypass correctly and he was in recovery and doing very well. Apparently, the bad bypass had been done at another VA, some states away. My cardiologist friend confided that he came closer than he ever had to telling a patient to find a good lawyer.

Curiously, this was the same patient whose wife called me in a panic one day sometime later, almost shouting: "He's up in a tree, sawing limbs, and he's been having chest pains. He won't stop and get down. HE'S GOING TO KILL HIMSELF AND MAKE ME

WATCH! WHAT SHOULD I DO?" I don't remember what I told her, but I'm sure it wasn't so great. What can you do? He didn't get down, though somehow didn't die. I thought: so much for our behavioral cardiology clinic and training.

Smoking Clinic

I inherited a smoking clinic from my former VA supervisor. I had rotated through the smoking clinic when I was a resident/intern, and so was prepared to walk right in when he took another job and I inherited his there at the VA. The clinic was designed to be a state-of-the-art (wish I could say "science") smoking treatment program to help veteran smokers referred to us by other medical wards. Some referrals were from vascular surgery, stating they would not do surgery until the veteran quit smoking (which was a major cause of their peripheral vascular–caused pain). Others came from cardiology, cancer, and pulmonary wards. All should have been motivated, but not so much. Many were two to three packs a day smokers who started during WWII or Vietnam.

I shouldn't have been surprised they didn't want or like the treatment. Ignorantly, we included in day one, a long education component showing all the disease and risks for smoking, including lurid black lung pictures, and diseased hearts and mouths. After that, they were given more education and set up for a rapid quitting schedule. They had to self-monitor multiple variables such as number of cigarettes smoked, when, where, and why, enjoyment levels, what they were doing, etc. When we looked at our results, we found our clinic dropout rate was 90 percent! They headed for the hills, often after the first session.

So, we—my team of clinical interns, colleagues (primarily Donald Prue), and research assistants—decided to start over. We threw out virtually all the educational components and the rapid schedule of quitting (allowing them to continue to smoke for a few weeks while we broke the habit down), and created the gradual step-down, brand-fading program[6] (later renamed for the public as the Smokefade program, using the same gradual approach to quitting). Sessions were changed to 10 minutes, and veteran smokers only had one new, small step each brief session. One session they were encouraged to change brands to a slightly lower nicotine-yield cigarette. We figured since it must have been nicotine addiction, why not fade them down slowly, brand-by-brand for a while and then step down to quit from an ultra-low brand that they weren't so in love with, rather than the higher nicotine-and-tar brand they so preferred. We also gradually disrupted and restricted the smoking habit by narrowing the window where they could smoke (we called it their "kennel"), and what they could do when smoking other than smoke. They were not allowed to do anything during that window, including watching TV, using the computer or the phone, eating, or socializing. All of these activities could serve as co-reinforcers for the smoking itself, and that was what we wanted to eliminate.

Further studies were conducted by my new team in a new university program[7], headed up by my top doctoral student, Christi Patten (who went on to a distinguished career at the Mayo Clinic Cancer Research Center of Minnesota). Christi co-authored and was lead author on a number of our scientific studies on treating smokers and evaluating treatment based on the fade-down program[8,9] and cognitive behavioral approaches with depressed smokers (many of whom are)[10].

Our new population of smokers included recovering alcoholics (about 90 percent of whom smoked) in our overall series of treatment studies[7-10]. At one point we had recruited, evaluated, and treated over 600 smokers through our state of California–funded research program (Project SCRAP-Tobacco—Smoking Cessation in Recovering Alcoholic Persons). We conducted these studies on our integration of the Smokefade and brand-fade program into 12-Step AA language (as well as some techniques such as the "Dear John Letter" (I resent that)—saying final goodbye to the habit that had been a great friend for so long).

> **CAN WE TALK?**
>
> *Urge Control.* In addictions treatment, we spend a lot of time talking about controlling urges. In smokers, it's the urge to light up and smoke. In alcoholics, it's the urge to go into a bar, pick up a bottle, and drink. In compulsive gamblers and pornography and sexual addicts, it's the urge to go to places to engage in those behaviors or to go online. These urges or desires can be so powerful as to be overwhelming—the only thing that can stop them is to engage in the desired but unwanted behavior. That's the belief, and there is a lot of truth in that. But not so fast.
>
> There are a number of ways in which these urges can be avoided, intercepted, delayed, distracted, or defeated. One helpful point of understanding is that most urges go away on their own within three to five minutes. Just toughing and waiting them out can help. AA says one day at a time, but also one moment and one choice at a time. It all adds up. We also teach something called the DEADS—to put the urge to death, by delaying (D), escaping (E), avoiding (A), distracting (D), and/or substituting (S) something for the urge to commit unwanted behaviors such as drinking, smoking, unhealthy eating, pornography viewing, etc. These can be learned and practiced. Our negative addictive thinking can also be "automatic"—and we call those ANTS, for automatic negative thoughts. These ANTS cannot be played with, they must be killed—kind of like when I set fire to a red ant mound (but with less disastrous results).
>
> Social support, such as calling or texting a friend when tempted, or even while engaging in the addictive behavior, can be highly effective—but when used consistently. AA meetings tell you: "It works if you *work* it." Indeed so.
>
> *Suggestion*: Practice the DEADS, killing the ANTS, and seeking social support for these unwanted behaviors. You will strengthen the resistance muscles in you, your mind *and* behavior. Don't give up. Many are successful at this. You can be too.

We found that our gradual reduction and habit breakdown program worked as well as some of the best programs at the time—roughly 50 percent to 80 percent quit rates post (10-week) treatment, and 27 percent quit at one year (the gold standard in smoking-cessation studies). The conventional wisdom (even to this day) tells us that smokers are addicted to nicotine; however, our studies indicated that it was much more the behavioral and social conditioning factors that controlled the behavior than nicotine—which is much more like caffeine in coffee in terms of its psychoactive effect on the brain and person. Withdrawal was also not as severe, common, or characteristic in our smokers who quit or cut down significantly. When it did occur, it was milder and more like behavioral and emotional withdrawal due to the disruption of a compulsive habit, such as a gambler who quits. In fact, most smokers quit all the time, on their own, when they are ready, and not so much through outside education or force (although that could help).

But our success attracted attention—both from the researchers and addictions treatment folks who opposed the "warm turkey" gradual fade-down or "harm-reduction" approach. It was "all-or-none" to them (including many in the government research and funding agencies)—and from some unwanted and unexpected sectors of the public.

A Smoking Gun
Unsurprisingly, we researchers and clinicians in areas such as smoking treatment are often consulted from the business world to help with things like evaluating and promoting their product, and that doesn't exclude attorneys hired by those companies. In fact, it was only relatively recently that the requirement was introduced to scientific journals that researchers disclose any and all associations and relationships, financial and otherwise, with the companies representing the products and services being researched or investigated. This also became an uninvited issue for me in my career as an addictions and tobacco and smoking treatment researcher, and it was a very difficult decision for me whether to "collaborate with the enemy" as it were.

My published reports and certain controversial findings led to my being contacted by attorneys for Big Tobacco. When I received the call, sitting at my smoking clinic building provided by my university and my large government smoking treatment grant, I laughed. "You must be kidding," I said to the attorney stuck with contacting me to try foolishly to convince me to represent them for expert testimony. Just about to tell him where to go and then hang up on him, I reminded him (they had obviously found and read many of my scientific publications on smoking treatment): "I've spent much of my career trying to undo the harm *your* clients have done. Thank you but NO THANK YOU."

But they talked me into at least letting them come out and take me to dinner and talk. They were definitely barking up the wrong tree, but I figured I could get a very nice dinner on their account when they persisted in wanting to come talk with me despite my well-directed curses at them.

At dinner, the three questions posed to me were: 1. Are all smokers addicted to nicotine, and unable to quit because of that addiction? 2. Are smokers in their addiction to nicotine identical or highly similar to cocaine and heroin addicts? 3. Do nearly all smokers have terrible withdrawal when quitting or cutting down on their smoking? And, a fourth question was offered as well: Do smokers who switch to lighter cigarettes end up smoking more cigarettes to maintain their nicotine intake?

My four answers: 1. No; 2. No (definitely not); 3. No; and 4. Some, but generally only temporarily—according to our large tobacco-related clinical treatment and assessment studies, data analyses, and overall findings—most published in major scientific journals. The attorneys then said they were only looking for a scientist, such as myself, who has research addressing those answers, to help with writing scientific reports and possibly testify if called.

We knew that telling smokers that they are addicts, will have horrible withdrawal, and great difficulty, or will likely fail at, quitting was counterproductive and counter-motivational. These messages fly in the face of motivation research and our in-the-trenches work attracting, motivating, and causing reductions in and cessation of smoking—especially in the most highly dependent smokers such as those in the VA and recovering alcoholic smokers—our two primary pools of smokers recruited and referred to us.

After much thought and counsel (and prayer) from trusted friends, I decided they were entitled to a balanced, science-based report, within careful limits, and agreed to help just so far. It was also a time when I was going through a marriage breakup and separation, and the extra income was helpful.

My clinical research colleagues on the "other side" were not in agreement with me despite our research findings, literature analyses, and treatment data. Unfortunately, their approach included the employment of counter-motivational "scare tactics" to bully smokers into quitting. These well-intended efforts were more likely to push smokers *away* from quitting, motivationally and behaviorally. Fear and threats almost never work, and usually backfire. There is also a well-known "reactance effect" in which individuals will strongly resist any attempts to usurp their freedom in deciding whether and how to change. Unfortunately, many of my colleagues in the field did not seem to appreciate this evidence-based "counter-narrative."

Dad and the Marlboro Man

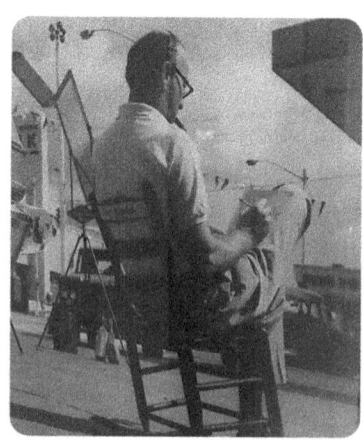

My father, the advertising guy, marketed lots of useful products, but also real disease—cancer, heart and lung disease—with cigarette campaigns. Here he is filming some kind of a commercial, maybe for an otherwise harmless product, but not the Camel cigarettes account, which he had. He never talked much about it, but my mother told me he helped to come up with the "I'd walk a mile for a Camel" campaign. I'm pretty sure it was through his contacts in the field of advertising, and probably tobacco marketing, that I was able to recruit the Marlboro Man creator, Jim Barnum, for a symposium I put together on health marketing. Jim was the head of the Ad Council, and (get this irony) the grandson of the great P. T. Barnum of the Barnum and Bailey Circus, who coined the "there is a sucker born every minute" storied declaration.

I recruited some well-known and published experts in tobacco control to present on the same symposium[11,12] as their "evil enemy," Marlboro Man Jim Barnum, and what a panel it was! Shall I say these other scientists and speakers (not to mention the prospective audience of treatment experts and addictions researchers) were not exactly good friends of Big Tobacco, or their "collaborator in crime" Jim Barnum. Would you believe, it didn't turn out so well? It didn't.

In my invite call to Mr. Barnum, I said I wanted him to talk about how they sold and marketed disease (I think I actually said that) so we could learn how to sell and market health using similar techniques. He humorously (but not entirely) accused me of wanting him to be a "sacrificial lamb on the altar of health." We both laughed, but it was true, and I pleaded guilty. Nevertheless, he accepted. I decided he was a brave man.

Anyway, Barnum gave a great talk leading us through the Marlboro cigarette campaign with the Marlboro Man smoking cowboys on their horses in the windswept great outdoors of the West. It was one of the most effective advertising campaigns ever, and especially in the tobacco field. He handled so gracefully all the boos, catcalls, shouts, and curses from the audience (*and* the fellow presenters, I'm remembering). Several times I had to step in, take the microphone, and attempt to quiet the outraged audience who were yelling at both him and me by that time.

Let's just say his talk and my chairmanship over the symposium were not exactly so well received by my health and medical colleagues and audience. I took a real "beating" (though Barnum, unlike me, was probably used to it and relatively immune from this sort of abuse). I later apologized to him on behalf of my field, myself, *and* my dad, though not many other representatives felt that same way. I'm pretty certain a plot was devised to run me out of the field after that, but it failed. Too bad.

But my enthusiasm for developing more creative and effective ways of treating the most highly tobacco-dependent smokers was ultimately stimulated, and I continue to the present day to work, entrepreneurial mindset-like, on the adaptation to the internet and website application of my successful Smokefade treatment program, for those most difficult smokers, using a cognitive behavioral and motivational approach, remotely *(smokefade.com)*. Thus far, it is promising but in need of a co-investor in order to refine and maximize its potential. By the way, might you know of anyone with deep pockets who might be interested? (Sorry, no referral fee, unless it is you.)

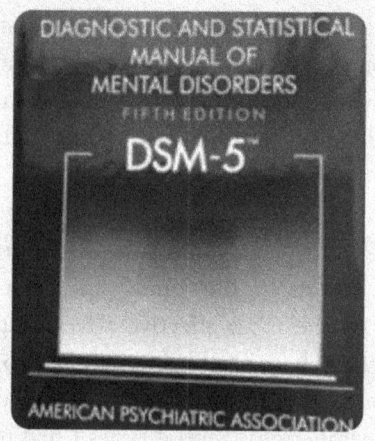

CAN WE TALK?

Barnum Statements, Psychological Gullibility and Personality Dis-orders.

P. T. Barnum was not only celebrated for his Barnum and Bailey Circus, but also for a notorious statement he apparently made about the gullibility and manipulability of the common person: "There's a sucker born every minute." His grandson Jim Barnum pointed out to me that this statement was taken out of context, and I never did find the whole statement, which I'm sure existed. But interestingly, P. T.'s sucker statement came into our vernacular even in psychology. We say that "Barnum statements" are broad, even nonsensical, statements that can refer to or describe everyone, and that we can use to fool, deceive, or manipulate people, and in psychological experiments where we often don't tell our subjects the whole truth, or any of it, to test reactions, deceptions, and responses.

A most interesting study that used Barnum statements had to do with personality testing of college students who were all given the same personality analysis after they took various tests to determine their unique personality traits. The personality profiles they all received made statements like: "You are a person who has many friends, but sometimes people don't like you" or "You can get frustrated with tasks and give up too soon, but you are a consistent and faithful person who almost always finishes what he starts." And so on. You get the idea. They were all Barnum statements. Here's the kicker: when these student volunteers were asked to rate the accuracy of their personality profiles with the Barnum statements, they almost always rated them as very accurate!

Personality "dis-order." Now don't get me started on all those Barnum statement-loving, hyper-psychologizing and categorizing-obsessed personality diagnosis folks (oh, I already have, haven't I). You know, those personality disordering, diagnostic "bounty hunters," and their companion crystal ball–gazing psychobabble spouters who try so hard to spot (or invent) your many personal psychopathologies, predict your behavior and your futures, your compatibilities and capabilities, you name it. Heaven forbid, if they had their way we will one day include a formal personality disorder diagnosis, say, by the 2035 DSM-10, with accompanying individual picture and life description, for every person in the world! Hey, everyone has a personality, so everyone must have their very own personality disorder. Their Diagnosis? - Let's just use their personal name. Wait for it. It's coming.

Compatibility. Have you ever looked for that "soulmate" with whom you are perfectly compatible? Maybe you've even taken tests together or individually and you "match." Consider this: there is core compatibility with things such as character, integrity, honesty, moral values, kindness, humor, gentleness, intelligence, and so on—pretty essential for a good relationship, and then there is the non-core, more peripheral compatibilities such as irritating habits, style of dress, politics (okay, maybe this is core), tastes in food, sports teams, and perhaps religious beliefs. The core compatibilities tend not to be easily changed, if at all, whereas the more superficial compatibilities can and do change. Thus, you are likely compatible in a relationship if the core values and characteristics are there and a close match, and not if you are not—the other compatibilities are not as critical.

Suggestion: Be careful about what you believe regarding all that people tell you about yourself or use to categorize or diagnose you. This may be particularly true for tests, programs, or analyses that use overly broad, generic (Barnum?) statements that could refer to almost anyone, and any future. Be particularly wary if they charge you for this "service" (can you say "astrology" and "palm reading"?). Psychology clinics and even church counseling centers can be guilty of it too. I've counseled individuals and couples who have been subjected to these kinds of overly general personality types, clinical diagnoses, and relationship compatibility ratings and predictions, and have had to spend time undoing the damage to their self-image, freedom of choice, motivation, life direction, choices of mates, or future directions in life. Maybe just stay away from all that stuff, trust your own heart, as well as those who know you best and love you, and perhaps God too.

ROOM 302

TRAINING TRAVAILS AND RESEARCH FUN

"Tell the truth and run."

—Yugoslavian Proverb

Psychiatry in Action Training Antics

While still a doctoral trainee, I had a crazy experience with a semi-hilarious, psychiatrist mentor. He was my favorite psychiatrist of all time, for whom I interned at a hospital affiliated with my doctoral university, and he was a character. Big old cigar in his mouth (smoking was legal and permitted in hospitals even back when) and a twinkle in his eye, he used to love to have fun with us. He would have been my psychiatrist if I could have afforded one then.

Would you believe he was one of these unusual physicians or clinicians who gave his home phone to all his patients?—even the crazy ones (remember he is a psychiatrist). He said they felt calm knowing they could call him if and whenever in trouble, and they rarely did. Amazing.

The psychiatrist (who will remain unnamed to protect his guilt) had a young kid at home and would regale us with stories of their time together, especially watching Mr. Rogers, which the doctor couldn't stand, but he loved his kid, and so watched. One day, perhaps with another twinkle or wink of his eye, he called us into a female patient's room and motioned for us to watch.

The woman was a catatonic schizophrenic, who could not speak or move. It's a type of psychological and behavioral "paralysis" characterized by repeated or relatively permanent catatonic, "frozen" states, or "waxy flexibility" in which an arm could be manipulated into position in space and would stay there. He took a syringe and injected something (it was sodium amytal, or "truth serum" we figured) into her IV line, and then began an audible countdown: "10, 9, 8, 7, 6, 5, 4, 3, 2, 1, 0." At zero, he asked the heretofore frozen woman a question and she immediately "came to life" on schedule at zero. They carried on a conversation for about five minutes. At about the five-minute mark, he looked at his watch and amazingly started the perfectly timed countdown once again, and at zero she lapsed back into her catatonic state as if on cue. I think he probably smiled and winked at us. I'm pretty sure he did. We stood heads shaking, amazed! Our favorite psychiatrist mentor was a bit of a show-off and we loved him for that. We hoped that she got better and were pretty sure our psychiatrist did everything possible to help her return to normal, or at least functioning.

Maybe you have heard this line making appropriate fun of psychiatry, and by proxy, psychology (I think my favorite psychiatrist would laugh with me):

"The neurotic is someone who builds castles in the sky.

The psychotic is someone who lives in them.

And the psychiatrist charges the rent."

Biofeedback without the Bio

One time our psychiatrist mentor referred a patient who had what was diagnosed as a conversion reaction—a psychosomatic condition in which he had a paralyzed arm. It was not actually paralyzed, as there was no organic reason for the dysfunction, but the patient believed it to be so, and so it was. The three of us graduate students decided to administer a biofeedback treatment for this patient. But it was biofeedback without the bio. (*Actual* biofeedback is a creation of psychology and physiological psychologists, *not* of psychiatry and medicine, as some of my M.D. colleagues sometimes contend.)

We hooked an analog meter to some lights, and strung electrodes from behind the screen hiding the polygraph or physiograph machine. But we could manually operate and manipulate the lights and meter. One of us put on the long, white lab coat and with a fake, thick German accent told the patient that when the electrical current was passed into his arm his arm would suddenly move and be healed. In reality, there was no electrical stimulation, only dead-end wires, but we didn't tell the patient. The imagined current "caused" his arm muscles to work and he was able to move his arm.

When we activated the meter needle and the lights, the "German doctor" commanded the patient to quickly move and raise his arm, which he fearfully did. "YOU VILL MOVE ZEE ARM OR ZEE MUSCLE MAY BE HARMED AND COULD EVEN EXPLODE!" Okay, maybe "explode" was not exactly used, but that was the message, and you get the point. Anyway: patient cured. We wrote the article up for the *Journal of Irreproducible Results*, a wacky science journal by goofy scientists (like us-to-be). I kept this citation on my CV for some time, but then wisely decided to delete it for fear of humorless faculty review committees.

CAN WE TALK?

Psychology vs. Psychiatry. Lots of people are confused about the differences between psychologists (like me) and psychiatrists, like my favorite cigar-puffing mentor.

The doctoral program I somehow made it into granted the Ph.D. degree, which means doctor of philosophy. The Ph.D. is the older and supposedly more distinguished academic, and more research-oriented, degree. The Psy.D. or doctor of psychology is the more recent addition, sanctioned and promoted by the American Psychological Association (the Big APA, after the smaller "little APA" of the American Psychiatric Association). The Psy.D. is generally considered the more clinical degree, and to be relatively equal in terms of clinical psychology practice and for many academic training programs as well. In programs that offer both the Ph.D. and Psy.D., the former is designed for those who want a more research and academic career focus, while the latter, Psy.D., is more for the person interested in clinical psychology practice, such as doing therapy and counseling, but there are exceptions at certain institutions that consider them equal for both specialties.

Many people are not aware of the differences between the psychologist and the psychiatrist. They are quite different in a number of respects. The basic difference, most have been told, is that the psychiatrist (a) has an M.D., or medical doctor degree, (b) follows the medical/biological/disease model (e.g., "find it, fix it"), and (c) is licensed to and does prescribe medications for treatment and "fixing."

The clinical psychologist, on the other hand, does not have and cannot legally (a) and (c), but adheres to the psychosocial/behavioral or health model of disorders and practices cognitive, psychodynamic, and behavioral assessment and treatment modalities. But both the psychiatrist and the clinical psychologist must be licensed in the state they practice in, usually after passing a written and sometimes oral examination before a professional board.

Finally, there are many specialists in psychological and behavioral therapies who do not have their doctorate and are not referred to as doctor, who have their master's degrees in either social work, psychology, or marriage and family therapy—primarily the LCSW (licensed clinical social worker) and the MFT (marriage and family therapist). These master's-level therapists, whose training is nearly entirely focused on clinical assessment and therapy, are often equal or superior to doctoral-level psychologists in the clinical therapy arena. Potential clients should consider these master's-level licensed therapists equally in their search.

A good friend, (Jeff W.) a psychologist who trained in the same internship class as I did, turned it around and made the distinction more favorable to us psychology guys: *The clinical psychologist (a) has earned the older, more distinguished Ph.D. degree, and (b) is trained to evaluate research and provide cognitive and behavioral treatments; and the psychiatrist does not and is not (a) and (b).* It was due to this difference in training and capability that the medical staff at the VA hospital typically requested a psychology, and not psychiatry, resident on call to the emergency department. Take that (gentle ribbing), my dear medical colleagues!

Finally, there is psychoanalysis. The psychoanalyst can be an M.D. psychiatrist (more likely), or possibly a Ph.D./Psy.D. psychologist, and conducts more intensive psychoanalytic therapy that is much more expensive and involves more intensive "treatment" oriented toward Freudian and neo-Freudian modalities. It likely consists of analysis three times a week or more for years. It has been criticized as being less evidence-supported and more fitting for those who are richer, have the free time, and are not so severely disturbed.

Suggestion: Be wise about choosing your therapy and practitioner. Check with others who have had successful therapy or counseling, look on the internet for reviews, and the American Psychological Association's "PsychologyToday.com" among other websites show bios and relevant information of a variety of professionals. Search on effective evidence-based therapies for the disorder or problem area you have, and do this research before finding your therapist—and ask him or her what modalities are used, how long it will take and what it will cost. Finally, if medication is mostly wanted or needed, the M.D. psychiatrist would be a better choice; whereas the psychologist or master's-level therapist who cannot prescribe would be best for cognitive, behavioral, and relationship therapy needs. Strongly consider those trained in either or (ideally) all of MI (motivational interviewing), CBT, EMDR (eye movement desensitization and reprocessing), DBT (dialectical behavior therapy), and FIT (feedback informed treatment)—each highly effective, clinically proven, evidence-supported approaches to therapy and counseling for a variety of problem areas. And don't be afraid to shop around and even try out different ones before you decide to stick with one.

From the Hospital Back to School

Having finished my pre-doc training (and crazy training travails), I then spent almost 10 years as a staff psychologist at the VA and

University Medical Center, from 1978 to 1987. From there, I went on to take a very different position, as an actual teaching professor on a university and medical school faculty.

In my new professional life there, I continued my work in smoking treatment and health psychology but expanded to community health interventions as well. It was a very different environment, and I had to adapt to new populations of non-hospitalized, healthier, younger people—students and community adults—with whom to study, teach, and conduct research.

Psychology was, in many universities like the one I joined, the most popular major—especially with women. By the way, why are female students called "coeds"? Coed was originally used when women began to be admitted to colleges and universities that became known as coeducational for the women co-'s.

So many of our studies are based on those most available subject populations—young, fairly normal and healthy, mainly white, and mostly female students, typically in psychology who receive extra credit for their participation. This would be what we call a nonrepresentative sample of people in general, but rather of those young, normal, healthy, more highly educated female students. Our study publications should always have a warning label, cautioning and maybe invalidating generalization of results to anyone else! But they don't—overgeneralization be damned!

Research Fun
There was research fun, of course (and why not?), with our student populations. One night, a coed subject was in our sound-deadened lab chamber, participating in a discrimination task to track by pressing a button at each beat (R-wave) of her heart. We were giving her feedback by having a light flash at each beat, and gradually dimming the light to dark, when we heard over the intercom, "Oh my God!... Oh my God!" Concerned, my fellow grad students and I got on the intercom and asked if she was okay, and what was the matter? She then exclaimed fearfully, "I think my heart has stopped!" Muffling our giggling, we recognized that when the heart rate tracking light had

gone out, she thought that meant her heart had stopped. "Your heart is fine and beating well. No worries, we've only turned the light out." Scary to her, but silly and humorous to the point of hilarity (hidden from her by the soundproof chamber she was in) to us lab assistants and would-be researchers.

Finishing a research project often required submitting data to one's professor on a tight schedule, and there was little wiggle room, especially for a dissertation experiment like mine. Oh, sure, I could have faked the data for the last subject who never showed up over my last weekend scheduled for the project, but of course I didn't. I had another more reputable and nefarious method. I went out on the street outside our lab and grabbed a random psych student as my last subject for my dissertation (bribing her with double extra credit for required research participation)—generalizability of results be damned once again!

Alcohol Research Fun

What better and fun place to conduct research than to study drinking on the university campus—not that drinking there was much of a common problem. But when a fraternity president in one of my teaching classes approached me with their alcohol issue, I had to say yes. This was one of those all-too-frequent occasions when one's own problem area has special research interest for the researcher (kind of like, you can tell what the pastor's personal issues are by tracking what he preaches on. Really. Maybe researchers too).

It was later on, when my drinking was no longer such a problem (you will see), and after I had discovered motivational interviewing/counseling approaches to problem drinking. It was a day while I was teaching on the topic of alcoholism when he asked me if I would come over and give a talk to his chapter on alcohol and drinking (they were on probation for wild parties, property destruction, and fighting—surprise, alcohol was involved). But I decided that maybe I could give more than a mere lecture, which wouldn't do much good, but to set up a program with my master's student collaborator, Scott Walters, using something called the "Drinkers' Checkup" or the "CHUG." The frat boys loved its title and they were *in*.

So, with Scott's help, we approached other fraternity and sorority presidents and ended up recruiting six Greek houses. We got research approval from our Institutional Review Board (IRB) to conduct the study to compare the effects of giving motivational feedback to the experimental fraternity and sorority houses, their drinking history, any problems in their lives related to alcohol use, how much money they were spending on alcohol (and what it could have bought them relative to the cost of a new car), their average and top level of alcohol intoxication, and alcohol-related problems, given their typical drinking episodes, etc. Then, I went into each house and conducted a live lecture going through their individualized checkup survey results. We did not judge that they had a problem; we were only there to discuss what they thought about their pattern of drinking and the results for them individually. They would decide what, if anything, to do about it.

Beer Guy
I would make my rounds around campus in the evenings to speak with those fraternities and sororities, generally when all were assembled for their regular house meeting, and I began to be noticed on campus. The first time I heard it, I didn't think it was for me: "Hey, beer guy." "That's the beer guy!" Looking over my shoulder for this guy, there was no one. Only me. Indeed, it was for me. I wore the title with pride. One day, I was about to begin my talk before a fraternity and a guy sauntered in late (holding a beer bottle, ready for consumption) and very nicely asked: "Is it okay if I drink this during your talk?" I think I laughed and deciding not to fight the inevitable, I said weakly but humorously, "sure." It was a good decision. No riot occurred.

Interestingly, Scott further developed the CHUG into the E-CHUG, that could be delivered over the internet, and it became one of the standard tools used by universities and colleges throughout the country as a first-pass intervention for students with drinking issues and problems[12]. Despite my encouragement to the contrary, Scott decided to donate it essentially to our university rather than making millions of dollars on it for the rights. I guess that is partly why he became a highly successful teaching and research professor and department head at a major university, while your very own professor beer guy is not.

More Research "Fun"—the Earlier Years

My illustrious past as a researcher started early on, ingloriously, as a new master's student in experimental psychology. As part of a graduate research course way back in 1971, I set up a study evaluating the reaction time differences in a digital (button-pressing) task, comparing students who had received a placebo (sugar pill) "tranquilizer" to those who received only a sugar pill. I wanted to find the difference between those who were told it was a sugar pill and those who were lied to (remember that deception in psychology experiments). Not surprisingly, those told they had received the "tranquilizer" had much slower reaction times than the control group. Big surprise.

Now before you get all authoritarian and ethical on me, this was before we had the formal IRB, Institutional Review Board and Ethics Committee, to approve all experiments—so nobody (me, that is) ever got in trouble after the department committee on research approved the experiment. To do such a thing these days would be criminal, not just unethical. Hey, we did make the experimental "sugar pill tranquilizer" group sit for more than an hour before letting them go home so they would not be "impaired" drivers or walkers. One student volunteer told us it was one of the best "highs" he had ever had.

Expectancy is such a powerful phenomenon in the psychology of us humans. Once my parents had a party in which they typically "spiked" the punch with plenty of alcohol. But each thought the other had done it, and there was none in the punch. Nevertheless, all the unknowing partygoers were most happy that night.

Even More Fun Researching—Exercise

I found another way to have fun and do research—especially in an area of personal interest and benefit—EXERCISE! It was a great combination as you will see.

Community Exercise Program for Those Who Hated to Exercise
I decided to create an exercise program in the community—to try to bring enjoyment into something many people don't find very much fun. This vision stemmed from a combination of my personal exercise routine (I was running marathons by this time); curiosity about how to apply behavioral interventions to develop and sustain the exercise habit; and my field of cardiovascular behavioral medicine, including my work with those with high blood pressure. It seemed natural to advertise to "those who hate exercise but know they need to exercise," and it was a popular community program that stimulated quite a lot of media attention, including my first TV interview.

So began a series of studies in which I evaluated the effects of a number of things. These included gradual behavior shaping (starting with just showing up the first day in exercise clothes and doing nothing more); the strategic use of verbal praise during versus after the exercise bout; and the differences between progressive time-related goals (brisk walking for 30 minutes) and distance goals (brisk walking or jogging one mile). My most devious but fascinating study included a forced relapse followed by reinstituting exercise using relapse-intervention methods. Could we get them to restart their exercise after stopping? This was study six in a series that was eventually published in a major scientific journal in clinical psychology[14].

When we introduced the requirement for this experimental group, that they completely stop all exercise for a 10-day period, you should have heard the complaints and whining from these former exercise haters! We had done such a good job (apparently) in creating the exercise habit that when we threatened to force them to relapse in order to test the methods for reestablishing the exercise behaviors, they wanted no part of it. But they'd signed up for the study and received and agreed to (remember this?) an informed consent. They were stuck! Know what happened?

Almost none of them returned to the next phase of the exercise program after their 10-day no-exercise period. They had to be included in the study as dropouts. Our conclusion, in our most objective scientific language: DUH! What did we expect? These experimental "subjects" attempted to instruct *us*, the glorified psychology researchers, in a basic motivation science corollary. Just like we know that people change when they are ready, willing, and (believe they are) able, people will also tell you (if asked, especially) what they are willing and unwilling to do. If they protest when asked to do something they no longer want to do, then respect that. We were young and dumb and on to the next experimental group.

Interestingly, when I went to publish the six-study series as a whole, the editor for the peer-reviewed journal argued strongly for dropping the sixth study that did not turn out. But I negotiated effectively, and we kept it in because of what did *not* work—an equally or more important finding. There are so many studies like this that are never published because they fail to support the hypothesis—often a critical "non-finding." By the way, do you research authors know that you can negotiate with journal editors about what you think is most important to include in your study, even if they do not agree? You can and should.

I had a close friend, running buddy (at conferences), and distinguished colleague named Ray, who had a rather brilliant strategy for getting his lazy graduate students to exercise and get fit so he could get much more work out of them. He had them wear their exercise (running mainly) clothes to bed that night, with running shoes placed at the side of the bed as well. They were not permitted to *decide* whether to go out on their morning run while in bed. They had to get up, put on running shoes, go out the front door, close the door, and *then* decide. Pretty smart. I think Ray got lots of work from them because his career flourished to the point of becoming the head of the 50,000-strong American Psychological Association.

I was also subject to this sort of nefarious exercise manipulation plan during my graduate school years by a so-called fellow grad student. Our (his, actually) plan was to meet at a local running track at 6 AM. He told me he would wait for me and not start until I got there. On those all-too-frequent, crack-of-dawn mornings I was not feeling up to getting up and running, I could not call him. He said he would not be carrying his phone, and I had to drive down to tell him I would not be running that day. Well, you know the rest. If I had to go to all the trouble of driving down there, why not run. I was already there. No fair. We have a psychological term for this mean intervention: antecedent (stimulus) control. No need to explain it, only that it worked to get me there to exercise with him. Still want to know? Okay, here's a poor attempt at an explanation.

> **CAN WE TALK?**
> *Stimulus Control and Habit Creation.* This is a method of inducing or stimulating a behavior using behavioral psychology. It is called antecedent control because it does or stimulates something *before* the desired behavior, and that causes the behavior or makes it more likely to occur. I used it for studying behavior when in graduate school, and later with our smoking treatment groups.
>
> Here's how I did it: I designated a spot for my studying behavior—my desk and chair in my apartment. I dedicated that place for studying only. Here is the powerful part: if at any point my mind began to wander, or the phone rang, I had to get up and leave that place. You can imagine at first how many times I had to get up and walk away. But eventually (maybe a couple weeks later after many trial periods), I was able to study nonstop without mind wandering for two or three hours at a time. It worked. I had shaped the behavior and developed the study habit. Here's the coolest part: since that stimulus of the desk and chair was conditioned to be associated with only studying, if I did not feel like studying but needed to, all I had to do was go and sit down in that spot and I not only felt like it but began to do it.
>
> *Suggestion:* Use this method to create and maintain a behavior you want. It's habit training or conditioning. Try it on yourself and in other areas, like eating (dieting) or smoking. Designate your place for the behavior, restrict it to only there, and do nothing other than that in the place. You can control your eating and your smoking should you want to cut back (and who wouldn't) by avoiding that dedicated place. For study, you want to go there. For eating and smoking, only go there, and only eat or smoke,

> and then leave. Got it? Of course, you do. It can work but may take some time (and practice!) to develop the conditioned stimulus for the behavior and the associated habit. Practice makes perfect!

Exercise for Hypertensive Seniors—Project HELPS

Another area of research for me was an extension of my personal and professional interest in exercise—applying it to the treatment of hypertension or high blood pressure. Submitting research grants in this area, I was fortunate to be funded for two major studies—one through the National Institute on Aging of the NIH, and the other in the VA for veterans with hypertension. In both studies, we found a significant beneficial effect of both aerobic (very brisk walking) and isocaloric (same number of calories burned) non-aerobic exercise (slower walking) in seniors with medicated high blood pressure[15,16].

Importantly, our blood pressure reductions, due to the exercise regimens, were equal to or greater than those from the medication. In one study, we were able to publish in a major peer-reviewed medical journal, and the other showed results that were "too good to be true." Our blood pressure reductions were so significantly better than anything that had been shown before with respect to exercise effects—especially including a study replication we conducted in South Africa—we decided to only present the data at national conferences but did not attempt to publish[17]. This was one of my greater disappointments as a researcher, particularly for the amazing South African results (with black Africans, who have a much greater mortality from hypertension than whites), as the data could not be retrieved and validated.

One of my more interesting presentations of those outstanding findings was at a special symposium at my medical school's department of physiology, run by one of the most distinguished medical physiologists in the world—Arthur Guyton, M.D., author of a medical "bible," *the* textbook for medical school training in medical physiology. I was especially interested in Dr. Guyton's take on our study data, thinking he would be able to talk as the top expert in the field of the physiology of hypertension and solve some of our questions about the mechanism and such of our powerful effects. Yet, curiously, he was most interested in how in the world we got those men to exercise! I think my answer was something along the lines of "Well, that's what we psychologists do, shaping and reinforcing behavior, no matter the task or difficulty." He never did tell me his theory of why we got such significant blood pressure reductions. He would have told us it had to do with the effect on the kidneys (you medical folks will know what I mean here—a colleague of mine once quipped that Guyton, "Mr. Kidney," believed the soul resided in the kidneys).

Research Exercising "Headaches"
Two final research fun episodes included studies we did in the area of exercise effects (surprised?) on headaches in a veteran with severe tension headaches, as well as with five women with debilitating migraine (vascular) headaches.

Study One
He had chronic headaches that affected his marriage and family especially, and the pattern intrigued us because normal relaxation training did not help (it almost always does in the case of muscle tension headaches, which he had). The problem was when he was not sitting still and relaxed, the headaches would come back. Therefore, we decided to train him to relax *while* walking and moving on a treadmill and hooked up to electrodes measuring and providing feedback on his muscle tension around the forehead and back of the neck. Producing relaxation in the muscles around the head and neck is a highly effective treatment for muscle headaches like he had.

The intervention worked great! His headaches went away, and so did he, a satisfied customer. But wait. He came back shortly thereafter. It did not fix all his headaches. He still had them, especially on the weekends. Strange, we thought. So we reassessed him. If I give you a hint—an important sign—do you think you could diagnose the problem? He was a long-haul trucker, working through the week, but not on weekends. What do truckers do to keep awake on long-haul driving? They drink coffee (and he definitely did—about 15 cups a day on average!).

Come to find out he didn't drink coffee on the weekends. Got it yet? You better. He was in caffeine withdrawal over the weekend! We then added the intervention of caffeinated coffee fading, gradually to decaffeinated coffee every third cup, and that did it. Weekend headaches gone too! We got this study published in the journal *Headache* for its creative clinical treatment[18]. Well done, Tim and Abby!

The second research project was done by one of my "good" interns (just kidding, they were all pretty good, and some great, like Jim). It was his doctoral dissertation, as it turned out, in which an aerobic exercise intervention was implemented with five females with migraine headaches. A delayed baseline design was used in which the exercise intervention was progressively delayed, subject by subject (a variant of the "n of one" single subject designs), to determine the effect of exercise across the series of those five patients. The results were positive—in four of the five patients, the aerobic exercise was found to significantly decrease or eliminate their headaches, and this successful study was published in a prominent scientific, behavioral psychology journal[19]. Nice study, Jim!

Jim's headache treatment study was what we term an "n of one," or N=1 study, in which you systematically apply a single, or multiple interventions, following a period of baseline tracking (A), and evaluate the effects of each treatment or intervention (B, C, D…) as compared to the baseline A. This has been called a case study or AB experimental design, which can be strengthened by subtracting and then reinstituting the treatment (B), to an ABA or ABAB design. This can be powerful evidence, especially if it is replicated over and over by multiple subjects with similar results showing bi-directional control of the targeted variable (for example, a medical disease or behavior). This is a legitimate scientific study, albeit much less controlled than the larger controlled, randomized group designs. I get frustrated when even people who should know better—like physicians and psychologists—call a large series of N=1 studies "anecdotal." These case-controlled studies produce legitimate evidence and are not anecdotal.

The Other Side of Research Fun—The Editorial Process
There is another side of research that you are likely not aware of that has an even greater chance of either promoting or distorting the accepted body of evidence than by the anecdotalists and horse-blinders-wearing-idiot "science" interpreters, and agenda-driven media and politicians (!): the secrets of the research literature editorial process! (Do not tell anyone I revealed the following to you. It is generally a well-kept secret in scientific and publication circles, and I would be in significant trouble if it were to be known I shared this with you. Thank you for keeping mum on this—especially on whom you heard it from.)

My career as a behavioral researcher included serving on various editorial boards of scientific journals. My role was an ad hoc study reviewer for these journals, and finally an associate editor of a major behavioral psychology journal. Interestingly, I was on the *other* side of the negotiation with respect to acceptance and publication of others' scientific studies. In that role, I selected the reviewers and made the final decision for acceptance or rejection of the paper, which may have included requesting or requiring a revision and even additional data analysis if I liked the study enough, but still had concerns. It was very unusual for a paper or study to be accepted outright without revision, but it does happen. Nevertheless, I didn't always gain the favor of my colleagues in the field when rejecting their papers and studies for publication. It went with the territory.

Two things about the role of the associate or "action" editor. First, if an associate editor at the journal to which you've submitted likes your study (or you), then he or she is more likely to assign "simpatico" reviewers (sometimes up to five but at least three, typically) who are more likely than not to give a positive review. We editors know who and who not to select, depending. On the other hand, if the associate editor does not like something about the paper or study (after reading it, presumably), then he or she might choose the meaner reviewers—those who love to find everything wrong and to say it in a not-very-kind fashion. The reviews and the associate editor's decision letter would then be sent back to the submitting (usually lead) author.

Second, the head or senior editor could do the same. If he or she loved the study or paper, it might be assigned to one of the gentler associate editors (if they exist), similar to the reviewer choices, and vice versa if it was not liked. I was never sure which category of associate editor I fell into. I could be pretty rough on authors, studies, and papers I did not like, but I could also be a pretty nice guy (can you say, "Barnum statement"?). Usually, the senior editor had final say on studies that were of particular interest and could veto decisions made by the associate editor. That happened only once in my term.

It was a study in which the investigators used a behavioral intervention, including biofeedback, to stimulate and modify the responses of an unresponsive patient who was in a vegetative coma. By definition, and medical diagnosis and condition of the patient, this should have been impossible. But according to the investigator's data, it was not: there was an apparent effect, and if true would have been an astounding finding. But mean Dr. Martin didn't like the science used, and my four reviewers were split on whether to accept or reject it for publication. So I rejected it (but with a highly laudatory letter—maybe like that rejection letter to the Korean student who came for orientation anyway—and maybe with some of those Barnum statements again).

But then the main editor stepped in. He very gently, but with persuasive wording, encouraged me to reconsider my decision and to submit it to new reviewers for a second look. I got the message. So I did. I believe we accepted the paper after all, but this was a long time ago, so don't ask me to search for and find it in the old copies of the journal I kept during my time as editor.

Were you aware that many legitimate scientific studies are never accepted for publication because they either did not show a desired or expected effect, or they disputed some so-called scientific consensus? Here's a private story that really happened and further emphasizes my cautioning us about the publication "politics" we face in trying to weed out non-science from legitimate science and "non-results" that should have been published to tell us what *doesn't* work (like my sixth community exercise study that the editors tried to "kill" but I wouldn't let them!).

My colleague, a quite well-known and well-published research professor at a major medical school, once shared his experience in reanalyzing some published data of a major medical research study. But his analysis resulted in a nearly opposite interpretation of the published result. When he wrote up his paper disputing the previous, improperly interpreted study, the chief editor of this major science journal—while agreeing that my colleague's analysis and interpretation was correct—refused to publish the new contradictory analysis. This journal editor said something along the lines that he would not publish it because it would be counter and too disruptive to the conventional wisdom that was already incorporated into the latest treatment of people with heart disease. Go figure (and beware).

The moral: there are negotiations at every level in science, not just between authors and editors, and particularly at the final stages of publication. So beware of all that you read regarding scientific consensus (no such thing) and with respect to what is true and not true. (You heard it here first.)

ROOM 303

WORLD-TRAVELING PROFESSOR

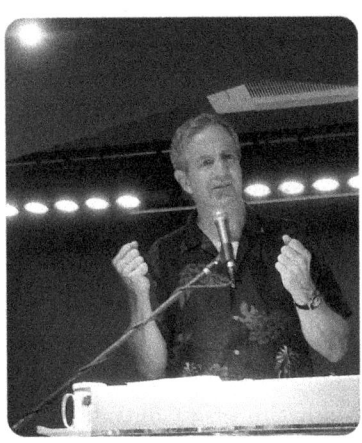

"Life is extinct on other planets because their scientists were more advanced than ours."

—UNKNOWN

The Traveling Professor

I found pretty early in my adult years that I loved adventures, especially while traveling around the world. In my professorships, I had the opportunity to teach, give professional presentations about my research, and actually conduct health-related and community research in several countries, including Australia, Canada, Eastern Germany, Southern Africa, Uganda, and South Korea. But I fell in love with Africa—ironically since one of my first prayers was to tell God I would go anywhere except Africa (I'll explain that in a later chapter). What's that they say about God? If you want to make God laugh, tell Him your plans. Indeed.

Sabbatical Travel

I was invited for three teaching sabbaticals over my 25-plus years as a professor—South Africa and Germany in 1994, and then South Africa again in 2001. The sabbatical in Germany took place not long after the Soviet Union collapsed and the Berlin Wall came down in 1989, and the sabbatical in South Africa, not long after their first free election in 1994. I then joined the US NIH team traveling to South Africa in 2003 to help with the AIDS pandemic, which at the time was worse there than anywhere else worldwide. I found to my pleasant surprise that English was their default language out of the eight native and Afrikaner languages. My love for the South African country and people led to seven more trips there after my initial one in 1994, on teaching, research, and church mission ventures.

My travels to South Africa started with those two teaching sabbaticals, first to Rand Afrikaans University (later renamed to non-Apartheid, University of Johannesburg after the election in 1994), and then to the Stellenbosch University, outside of Cape Town. My time teaching there was filled with exciting adventures meeting, teaching, and falling in love with the wonderful students and university staff—black, colored (an acceptable term there for mixed race), white, and Indian—who once took me on a walking tour of Soweto near Johannesburg that was most dangerous for a white man such as myself. The University wanted to send me there with an armed police escort, but fortunately the students warned me not to do that (saying it would "draw their fire") but to let them lead me there under their "protection."

The walking tour through Soweto (for South West Townships—their word for slum) was so amazing. I was the only white face among thousands of African blacks (my student tour guides and "protectors" were black); my nervousness was allayed when they found out I was an American. They expressed their gratitude for our government's leading support of the world's boycott of the South African white government that helped to bring it down and led to the free elections.

I was the rare American "hero" that day and couldn't help but feel the love and unearned admiration of many South African blacks there in Soweto. I was introduced all around and was honored to be a kind of "celebrity." I enjoyed the tour and meeting so many, not to mention the many offers of nasty sorghum homebrewed beer.

I was warmly welcomed by the students at the mainly white university, though there were clearly a number of black and colored students there, including my tour guides. I think it got as high as 20 percent black and colored soon after my first trip. A second sabbatical seven years later led me to a university in Stellenbosch, near Cape Town, which introduced me to many more outstandingly friendly students and professors, and especially townspeople involved in church ministries serving a poor township in their area. My third trip to Southern Africa was for my work with HIV and AIDS on a US NIH grant that I will describe later.

I had a wonderful friend and colleague named Ed, who was South African. We went through our doctoral training program together. He was one of those brilliant people who could rote memorize things after only seeing them once. It made me jealous, or at least envious, of how easily he seemed to dance through all those impossibly hard courses. It was at his behest that I was invited to South Africa for my first of three sabbaticals, some years before I was included in the US NIH HIV/AIDS team to that wonderful country.

Ed visited me in San Diego one year and I'll never forget his comment when I suggested we go visit our world-class zoo: "John, we LIVE IN A ZOO! Why would we want to come to visit yours?" Point made. It would have been like the "busman's holiday" in which the bus driver takes his vacation riding on buses. On one trip seeing him there, he was caring for more than a hundred clients. I had *no* idea how he did that until when driving around his city there in South Africa I found he was on the phone almost constantly with one of his reported 500 (!) clients. I wasn't so sure how one could counsel so many competently and ethically. But if anyone could have, it might have been my brilliant friend and colleague Ed.

Rita

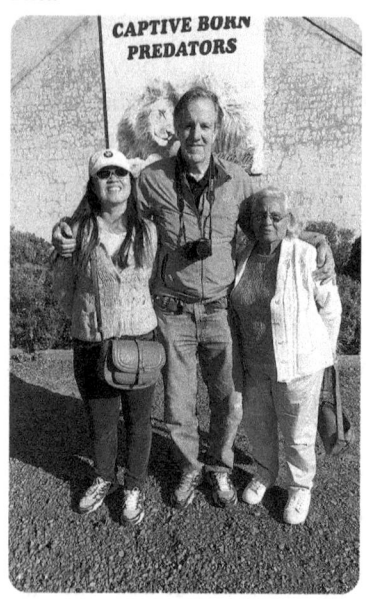

Then there was my Auntie Rita, a diminutive colored woman who became a dear friend and auntie of mine. Here she is on one of my recent visits to South Africa, with my wife, Catherine, and me. I was introduced to her by one of the colored students I was working with at the university, and she had a very "exclusive" bed and breakfast apartment in her home up in the colored section of the town. She became my auntie soon after we met. She loved to talk, and I was a good listener (you actually had to be around dear Rita). My next several trips to South Africa, including when I brought student research assistants with me, were punctuated with visits to Auntie Rita and her beautiful little place up on top of Stinkhout Crescent, by the road to Franschhoek. It became and still is my second home there.

Rita worked and lived for a time in Canada and London but was South African through and through. Born and raised there, she had many family members living close by and I think I met all of them, including at one of their legendary *braais* (their barbeque parties where they grilled wild, very tasty meat sausages mainly). She descended from the very short Hottentot people, described by Michener in his classic novel of South Africa.

Rita and I became so close, she would refuse charging me for my stays there, no matter how long (some more than a month), but we compromised on my bringing her favorite expensive French perfume, which I would buy on the trip over at an airport duty free. She was surprised the last time I visited when I remembered and came packing you know what.

I truly had fallen in love with the people of South Africa, and really Africa in general, and Rita holds one of those special places in my heart. By the way, did I tell you she was older? During my most recent trip there, where my wife and I stayed with her (no charge, she once again insisted), she was 86! She looked 60 and was one of those high-energy "whirling dervish" people you have probably met. Her "whirlingness," by the way, included her love of talking in that high-pitched British accent she obtained from Capetonian and London time growing up and working. But sometimes she would wear you down, so my wife and I would tag team it, taking turns listening to this precious lady and auntie.

The Salvation Army—South Africa
While over in South Africa for the sabbatical at the university outside Cape Town, I connected with an amazing program for the treatment of alcoholics and drug addicts—the Salvation Army Rehabilitation Program. I went with a colleague from my university who accompanied me on that trip to visit this program. It was located in the beautiful countryside in the wine farm area (some of the top wines in the world are from this region of South Africa, after the French Huguenots came down there centuries ago to escape religious persecution and brought their wine industry as well). At this rehab program—the only private residential program available at no cost to the desperately poor blacks and colored clients who were otherwise dying of their addiction—their residential clients worked the farm and attended meetings, generally staying for a year or longer. But some were too sick and eventually died from the ravages of alcoholism on their bodies and spirits.

On several of our visits, we got to tour and interview many of their program residents and the loving staff that devoted their lives to helping these desperately poor and sick men. Importantly, the residents we talked with pointed to powerful religious conversions that turned their lives around, and the army captain reinforced this core component of life transformation: God and His Spirit. Our hearts were so powerfully touched that my colleague and I kept in contact with them even after returning to the States.

Clearly, alcoholism was and is a huge problem in South Africa, especially this wine region in which the field workers were paid with wine or used their pay to purchase wine with vouchers (called the dop system—for a "dop" of alcohol—made illegal by the government but still practiced "under the table" too often). They would often work all week, then on Friday night buy all their wine and alcohol and be drunk all weekend. It was not unusual to see many drunk men on the street corners every weekend in town. Many of these men and women were dying not only of alcoholism but of "tik" (methamphetamine) addiction as well. Not surprisingly, South Africa is also the world's leader in something called "fetal alcohol syndrome" or FAS, in which babies born of alcoholic mothers suffer a form of brain damage, characterized in part by identifiable (flattening) facial abnormalities.

More Africa

Later trips to my beloved Africa included Namibia, Swaziland, and Uganda in central Africa. My Uganda trip consisted of a two-week stay for a training workshop to help psychiatric nurse practitioners learn motivational counseling for their work with the most seriously mentally ill, specifically for problematic medication adherence and behavior change needs.

Sitting in my room upon arrival the first night before the training conference at the major psychiatric hospital in Kampala, where the conference was taking place, I recognized a most beautiful song coming from the conference room below. So, I headed down there and found myself in the midst of a stunning church service—where most all the nurses at the conference were worshipping God. I walked in, only white face in that sea of beautiful spiritual blackness, sat down (to the surprised and welcoming looks of the all-black congregation), and enjoyed church with them. The two weeks of training went so well after that. They were wonderful, attentive, professional "students" whom I came to admire so greatly for their amazing commitment, hard work in impossible circumstances, and their necessary toughness and love.

Some years before my Uganda trip, my introduction to Africa was my first sabbatical originally scheduled for 1984. It was just before their election and turnover of the government from white rule to democratic (black) control. But I was told *not* to come because they were expecting a "blood bath" revolution, and white people would not be safe. I rapidly changed my plans, not wanting to "waste" my sabbatical approval from my university.

East Germany

Through a colleague's contacts with Germany, I was able to arrange a stopgap teaching sabbatical at one of their graduate schools, and so off to Eastern Germany with my wife and four-year-old son I went. While there, I taught in English, fortunately because I spoke not a word of German (I did know *ja* and *nein*, of course, as well as some English words usurped from the German, like "kindergarten" and such). Many of those once behind the Soviet Iron Curtain before its 1989 collapse spoke little English—at best it was their third or even fourth language after German, Russian, and maybe French—but they wanted me to teach in English (good thing because I spoke none of their other languages). They were for the most part enthusiastic and very friendly students, some even close to my age.

It was most interesting to me, though, how formal they were, especially in addressing their traveling American professor. I was a little embarrassed to be referred to as "Herr Doktor Professor Martin." Wow, three honoring titles. I liked it the more and more I heard it. (I thought I must start demanding that from my American students once I get back.)

I connected pretty strongly with two students, whom I subsequently invited and brought over to the US on an internship paid by their school—to attend my classes at home and participate in my research. I fondly remember one young man named Stephan. When I first asked the German class why they wanted to take a class from this American professor, he loudly proclaimed: "Because I LOVE

America! I want to BE AN AMERICAN!" I came to love this young man and his passion for my country, though I couldn't say I shared his view as entirely and as passionately as one who knew lots of her faults too. The other was a wonderful Hungarian woman named Jana, who became an even closer friend, and we maintain periodic contact to this day.

Korea
Some years later, in 2008 or 2009, and now on the faculty of a graduate school of psychology at a theological seminary, I was invited to speak in South Korea. My trip there was to present a two-week workshop on motivational interviewing and counseling to a graduate seminary in Seoul. I found the culture there fascinating, and the bustling capital city vibrant, if not super crowded when I tried to walk through their markets, shops, and incredible underground subway train and mall system. Unlike years before in Germany, I found that I was a head taller (at 6'3") than most of the Koreans on the streets and markets and could easily see over them. But the language was still an issue as most of the middle-aged and older Koreans spoke little or no English, and the young Koreans who did were not much interested in talking to me. Because the US had around 50,000 troops still stationed in Korea, I would regularly see small groups of GIs on the sidewalks and especially on my trip up to the DMZ, the highly militarized border with North Korea.

Entertainment for me, when not being invited out to dinner by my hosts, included watching South Korean soap operas on TV (I became a real fan) and learning to eat and actually like kimchi with hosts who invited me out to local restaurants (it's an acquired taste, but has been said to keep the SARS virus from China at bay). For the Korean TV soap operas, you didn't really need to know what they were saying in Korean to figure out what was going on. You know, family and relationship dramas are universal. I also found that I could go to the movie theater for the many American films that were not dubbed into Korean (they were often subtitled in Korean). I could figure out what was going on more quickly than those reading the subtitles—with comedy especially. I would get the joke and laugh out loud seconds before the Koreans could read and understand the writing and then laugh. That was fun.

What was more curious was my teaching alongside one of my graduate students—a South Korean woman (Priscilla Sihn)—who translated for me. Even though many of the students I was lecturing knew English, they didn't know the psychological lingo, and so translation was needed. Funny, but I noticed that what I said in English, stopping for translation, gave rise to a much longer series of sentences (paragraphs even) in apparent Korean (what did I know). This graduate student of mine knew the subject so well, after my fantastic teaching and mentoring of her, that I realized she was correcting, improving, and even simplifying what I'd said so the students could better understand. I think I eventually told Priscilla (her chosen American name) to explain this or that to them—trusting her to do a far better job than I. She did a great job. I'm wondering if the students, hearing my simple "tell them about what this means or how this works" or "explain this exercise to them" thought, "Wow, English is *so* rich and effective a language that it only took that one sentence to mean *all* that in Korean!"

Another international application of my training in motivational communication happened on a trip to Romania. It's one of my favorite stories. See if you agree.

Romania

It was just after our 9/11 tragedy, and our ministry team was invited to Romania, which was still suffering the ravages of decades of fascist and then communist rule. Romania had been one of the richest countries in all of Europe. I remember flying over New York City, my birthplace, and seeing two grieving plumes of smoke drifting skyward above the two fallen towers.

"Martin, you go"—to give a lecture to high school students on (the evils of) drugs and alcohol. They all agreed. I was the one psychologist on the mission trip, needing to be thrown to the wolves, and the Romania mission group was pretty convinced that I should convince those high school students about the evils of drugs and alcohol—a huge problem in their new "freedom." We were there to support a Christian ministry and church in a city outside Bucharest and were asked to go talk to the students at a public school as one of our (my!) "appointed duties."

It was a *trap*: A bunch of high schoolers, and *I* was going to lecture and convince them *not* to use alcohol and drugs for pleasure? I wasn't looking forward to it at all. So I decided to throw them a "curve." It couldn't hurt, and there certainly wasn't anything to lose. I remembered a technique I had learned but never tried some time ago during my training in motivational interviewing and counseling. It was time for the reverse debate, paradoxical intervention.

When I was led into the room with the students, expecting to see just a classroom of maybe 20 kids, I was taken aback to find the classroom was an auditorium, and the 20 students were about 300! I dove in headfirst, hanging on for dear life to my training in motivational communication. "What do you all think about alcohol and drugs?" I was not quite ready for the flood of shouted positive stories, joy-filled praises, and funny experiences that accompanied their sharing. I began by praising them for their great participation and detailed information, carefully and fully reflecting what they were saying and meaning (reflection), and regularly putting reflections together in common themes. After my final summary to the big group, I said I had an idea about doing something that would be fun, if they might like me to tell them about it. Of course, the answer was a loud, communal yes!

So, I explained that I wanted to have a debate with them—an argument even—if they were brave enough to try to outdo me, since I was a great debater and would be very hard or impossible to beat. Well, you can imagine the response to that. They were ready, willing, and able, indeed. Then I asked them who was the leader in the class—who might be the best debater. Many pointed to this one guy, and I invited him to come forward as I positioned two chairs opposite each other. Reluctantly, he came up to the stage, with much encouragement from the many students. Then I pulled the "switch." *The paradox.*

I explained that I was going to argue *for* why drugs and alcohol are a good thing, and he was to argue for why they were *not* such a good thing. Well, you would have thought he was a deer in the headlights. He just stared at me, speechless. With some coaxing from me and the students (after their shocked and then delighted laughter at the "switcheroo" I just pulled), he seemed to nod, and then I jumped in, summarizing what I had heard and making a strong case for why they were so great and no big problem. I said: "Your turn."

He began timidly, until I told him he was going to have to be *much* tougher on me if he was going to win this argument! So, I invited all the students to help him as well. At that point the shouting of all the reasons began (many quite good that I might not have thought of had I been lecturing). We went back and forth, and with the students' help he became better and better at passionately arguing for why drugs and alcohol were or could be a real problem and not such a good thing for them.

After about 15 minutes or so (I forget how long, but it seemed to be a longer time than it must have been), I began to slowly be weakened in my arguments, and even kind of talked into considering his/their more and more cogent arguments. I then summarized all that had been said on both sides, weighing their arguments with more strength and detail. I then asked them all to vote on who won. I don't have to tell you how they voted—with vigor—against *me*! I finally thanked them for the lively and fun time with them, excused myself, and left. I knew that maybe their own arguments had affected even a few to reconsider the goodness of drinking and using drugs from the discrepancy-enhancing change talk and arguments for change that occurred that afternoon. It was an experience I've shared with many, to their delight usually, and I'm sharing it now for others who might have an opportunity to influence in loving and effective motivational ways.

Back to South Africa (Again): The AIDS Epidemic

I was honored several years after my first trip to South Africa to be selected as the lead (okay, truth and reconciliation time: I was the only) behavioral scientist by NIH/NIAID to travel with the first special US team to help with South Africa's HIV/AIDS epidemic. My role was to train a variety of medical and other professional and lay workers, military as well as government civil servants, including physicians, nurses, counselors, pastors, and workers, in motivational interviewing and counseling. In particular, the training involved working closely with those learning how best to counsel people with HIV or AIDS for medication compliance and lifestyle change.

Most importantly, this was a time in South Africa when their post-Mandela president and health minister were blocking efforts within their country and throughout the world to declare the epidemic as mainly sexually transmitted, and to allow medications to be distributed to those infected. Because the South African Defense Force were losing many of their soldiers and family members to AIDS, they went around the obstruction of the health minister by declaring a military crisis and sought a military solution. Their generals approached the US NIH, and America wanted to help, which involved forming the training team and donating medications for the fight.

South Africa soon was recognized as the world's leader in HIV transmission and AIDS deaths, primarily due to sexual transmission between homosexuals and heterosexuals, and between the two. So many were sick and dying that the main social event in the poorest neighborhoods of the blacks and coloreds was the almost daily funeral processions. I was able to observe them as they marched and paraded through townships I was visiting and providing training in. It was like the New Orleans funerals with the somber and then celebratory band with horns and drums. Especially hard-hit were the black townships and many colored sections who showed HIV and AIDS prevalence rates between 25 percent and 50 percent (the latter in some Zulu populations and those of the Eastern Cape). Death and disease had devastated much of South Africa during my earlier visits and training there in the late '80s and '90s, especially before widespread use of the antiviral medications brought at long last to the country.

It was such a pleasure to work with groups of these doctors, especially nurses, and other health workers, like the two special multilingual assistants pictured with me at an earlier visit to the Western Cape of South Africa. Vatiswa and her sister, shown here with me in the picture, provided tremendous assistance in helping with translating effective behavior change and motivational strategies into the several languages of participants there in South Africa—critical to HIV prevention and AIDS treatment adherence. Thanks to a grant program, Vatiswa traveled to San Diego to stay with a mission family and attend classes and training work with me on the AIDS project from the US side. I lost touch with her and hope she and her sister are well.

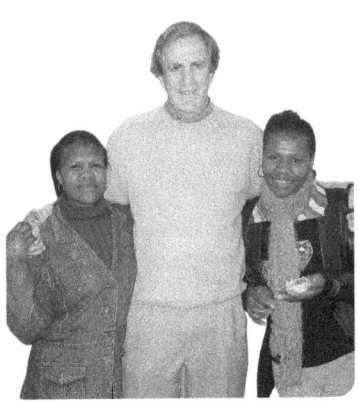

Despite my regular trips to Africa and training Africans in the HIV and AIDS projects, I was in culture shock, especially with regard to communicating with the wise African nurses. During one presentation by me in Namibia before a small group of nurses who worked with HIV-positive pregnant mothers, I ended up doing all the talking—not the best strategy when wanting to actively train and interact with people, especially from a different culture and society. For example, when I would ask a question or for feedback or questions on what they thought or had understood, I would wait a typical American pause (maybe five or ten seconds at most), and when there was no response, I'd move on.

One night, between daily sessions, I was approached (more like reproached) by one of the conference and training organizers. He told me I needed to recognize the big cultural difference in how these African nurses communicated. I was informed I needed to *shut up and wait* for them to process and respond in their normal time and fashion. So the next day I did. But it took lots of self-talk ("John, wait, wait, they are thinking, don't talk, they are processing, give them time.") and tongue biting. However, after what seemed like an age—really more like 30 or 40 seconds—their response arrived! The faces of these African nurses were apparently expressionless, that is, until I waited for and truly listened to their voices and wisdom. Then their faces transformed from both the appearance of coming to life and grabbing my heart. It was an incredible experience listening deeply to each of them as they shared. I could easily get lost in them and what I was experiencing from them—wisdom, gentleness, and peace. Amazing. I had no idea. It changed the way I presented after that, not only in Namibia, but also Swaziland.

Swaziland
My travels for training in motivational interviewing/counseling for nurses who worked with HIV-positive pregnant woman extended to a wonderful small country in southern Africa called Swaziland. I fell in love with the nurses there, and apparently they with me (they tried to get me married off to one of the King's yearly "Parade of the Virgins" who were not selected). My work with these nurses was similar to the work I did with the Namibian nurses. We discussed and trained in motivational styles of helping mothers choose between breast and bottle-feeding (HIV or other illness transmission risks for both), and adherence to medication and lifestyle change prescriptions and recommendations. The following is a copy of a journal entry from my time there.

CAN WE TALK?

A Taste of Beautiful Swaziland and Her People. I was profoundly touched by the stories from the nurse-sisters there in this beautiful land. I tried to get to know them in a better way, especially during breaks in my presentation, and before and after the day's agenda. I especially got to spend time with some locals and their goats.

An extremely nice and quite pretty young Swazi woman kidded with me in good English about entering the "Kingdom" with a true King. I asked at the border—will I get to meet the King? The officer didn't see my humor right away and said kindly that the King is all over the country and I might. My lady friend and local tour guide represented these attractive and extremely happy people, and their strong Christian faith. I see scriptures on the walls of homes like hers such as, "As for me and my household, we shall serve the Lord" of Joshua 24:15.

My host is named "Happiness" (Happy for short—surprise), and she tells me she is a "born-again Christian" when I inquire. I find out from another that the "old King" of Swaziland, maybe the current King's grandfather, had a vision of God handing him the Bible and telling him to follow it. He did, for the whole country, at least for a while.

The night before the training here in Swaziland, I was invited to a traditional *braai* (BBQ) at Happiness and Patrick's nice home. It was unbelievably tasty meats, sausage, chicken, and pork chops (can you say paleo diet?). I go back for seconds without coaxing. The next morning, I sit in the little restaurant at the hotel overlooking the most beautiful valley, mountains on both sides, green and lush with trees and plants. The training venue is also a little restaurant on the other side of town, with beautiful African architecture and a high-thatched roof, old wooden pillars, and African artwork around. The porches and decks out back overlook a really pretty stream and lush forest, rising to a large mountainside, green and lush. Such beauty.

The quietness and gentleness of the people here is striking, and I fall in love each day more with these nurses. The training goes well with my fellow presenters, Katie, the nurse, and Alan, an older hippy physician from Britain—both were dedicated to helping rural Africa through their terrible health crises including AIDS (Swaziland had among the highest prevalence of HIV and AIDS in all of Africa—a remarkably sad statistic). Dr. Alan, my fellow presenter, was married to a Zulu woman and living in South Africa.

The training conference at which we were to speak included all nurse-sisters (they call them sisters for some reason, which apparently means they are nurses and not necessarily Catholic nuns). Like Happiness, they were a people so humble, quiet almost to a fault (if that is ever a problem). In my new learning, I wait long periods after posing questions to them before anyone responds. The early pace of the training would have driven me crazy in my more American style of getting quickly on with things, but I watch Alan and Katie work slowly and effortlessly, and soon learn that this is relationship and group-building, and to hurry through this process would be so un-African and frankly ineffective. You don't rush through anything, much less these humble, quiet people. I notice a funny thing: the waiters are bringing pitchers of water with steam coming out of the top. The nurse-sisters are pouring and drinking what appears to be just hot water. I ask later and find that it is indeed hot water—apparently a common drink in these parts. I later find out it helps "cool" them somehow during the heat of the day (I found this very strange), and that they were all poor enough to want to save the money on paying for tea.

We sit out for lunch break on the rear deck to the sounds of an old billy goat (I find out later his name, get ready for this, is "Billy") baaaaa-ing. A baby goat follows him around the grounds. I mention this to the manager at the end of the day, and she says if we don't happen to see him tomorrow then we will know what happened to him (as she glances toward the kitchen). I laugh, but not too hard. Next day, no Billy. We had goat stew as one of the dishes for lunch. Quite aromatic and tasty. But I went

> out on a search for him today, and he was up in another field eating with his "girlfriend" Martha and her two little babies (actually called "kids!"). Cute. I was relieved that Billy was still alive. The very friendly young Swazi guy walked up with me to find them, and he taught me how to play with Billy—push on his horns and he pushes back. When I would jump at him, he would rear up, twisting his head like a mountain ram, and come at me. So, we played this for some time until my hands reeked of his unique scent. Phew.
>
> We start off with Christian prayer by one of the sisters (they don't so much ask if they can, but just do it as a natural start to any meeting). One time they asked me to lead. I was honored and did. Another powerful time was during an exercise talking to the group about their experiences counseling those with AIDS, and several talked with gentle but deep emotion and sadness about those patients of theirs who have died of this terrible disease. Many of us did not have dry eyes after listening to these heart-rendering stories of compassionate counseling and loving care.
>
> One day, Happiness asked the nurses there to sing a song and they all sang "Be Still and Know that I am God" in both Siswati (the language of Swaziland—much like Zulu to the south) and English. It was a moving and very beautiful moment for me, and as I read through this section during my editing review of the book manuscript, I find tears rolling down my face and my heart swollen with a deep sense of love and joy for that time and those special people and memories.

Zululand Pain

One of my most interesting, although personally painful, international research opportunities was my trip to Zululand near Durban, South Africa. If I had been a surfer (I grew up in the Northeast and Midwest, not much surf there), I would have visited one of the world's greatest surfing areas—Richards Bay—near there (sans great white sharks, of course). But after my training with physicians there in Durban on motivational interventions for HIV/AIDS patients, I was blessed (or so I thought) with a "thank you trip" to Zululand nearby. The Zulus were the mightiest tribal groups in Southern Africa (see some of the great movies and TV series on this, including *Shaka Zulu* and others), and their rich cultural heritage was all on display at the visitor center to which I was taken.

But I got to attend a ceremony while there in which the Zulu maidens, wives, and men all danced in their beautiful native regalia. It was both a fascinating and fun experience—that is, until my personal encounter with pain patient empathy (helpful, if not necessary, in working with the chronic pain patient like my time in the VA running that program!). It was an experience I couldn't—but should have—passed up.

The Zulus love to dance, and it was a delight to see the Zulu women and men perform. But this was not a place for the non-Zulu white guy researcher to accept the maiden's coaxing to step out of the visitor crowd and dance with the men. Beforehand, the unmarried maidens danced with nothing covering their upper body (one had to be sure to keep his eyes at head and eye level), and the wives were covered with beautiful bead necklaces. But the men's dance was quite unique and unknowingly dangerous. They had this high kick, straight leg to forehead, that I decided (here's the danger, plus idiocy) I could do too.

I don't remember if my kick actually got to my forehead like these limber and highly fit Zulu men, but that didn't matter the next morning when I rolled out of my apartment bed, hoping the university would notice I was not there, and they would call a doctor. Miraculously, they did (I couldn't even reach the phone), sent a local doc, and he gave me the most wonderful shot in the butt—a powerful anti-inflammatory and probably pain med that got me up and moving! Wonderful. I still visit that doctor when I make trips to my favorite second country. Nevertheless, I got a firsthand (or leg) look and experience with disabling pain—a condition common to a number of my patients in the hospital, veterans with PTSD, and many other clients. Compassion and empathy come the hard way some (or many) times.

FOURTH FLOOR

PSYCHOLOGY OF LIFE AND FAMILY LIVING

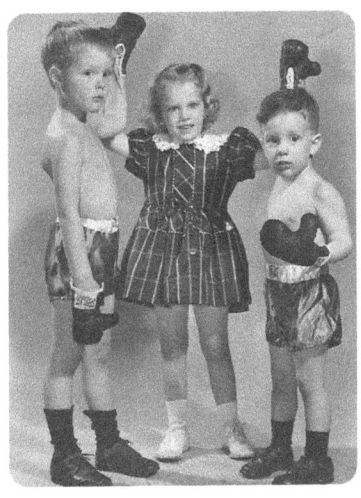

*"Nature or nurture.
Either way, it's the parents' fault."*

—UNKNOWN

Now we turn to the home and animal front, where in all honesty, we learn lots of psychology outside the classroom and research setting—in the *schools* of life and work. In my case, and perhaps in yours too, a wealth of things psychological came from our crazy families (from which I've already shared some stories) and those goofy animals as well—dogs and cats in particular. And I have got some stories, including more from my crazy time in that wonderful children's hospital as a special ed teacher, cutting my psychological teeth on the way in my wild career in the adult sphere. See if you relate to any of this. I think you might.

ROOM 401

ANIMAL PSYCHOLOGY

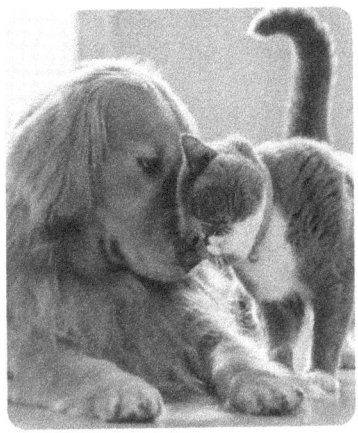

All dog/cat pair pictures provided by Animal Wellness Center of OC, Costa Mesa, Ca (animalwellnessoc.com)

"Animals are such agreeable friends—they ask no questions, they pass no criticisms."

—GEORGE ELIOT

I can't exactly take you for a tour through psychology without talking about animals, with our rich history of animal psych experiments and the animal psychology from the home front. It's a good time to do that, don't you think? So, here we go.

We learn a lot from our animals, not just in the experimental laboratory, but in that laboratory of the family animals. Come to think of it, child and adolescent psychology is a *lot* like animal psychology, and the family is a powerful, animal petri dish laboratory of learning. The principles are pretty much the same, and behavior is behavior, no? You parents will agree with me here: our kids can be a lot (too much?) like animals, behavior-wise that is, and sometimes in brute animal instinct ways.

Psychology has learned much about animals from behavior experiments, and as I say, from observing and working with kids and teens. My favorites are monkeys, dogs, cats, and I guess, pigeons, but there was that one bear that I will get to. Let me give a little background here. You might find this interesting, if not fascinating, which I did, of course.

From Kids to Animals

So are we in agreement, my fellow parents, child psychologists, and psychiatrists, that kids are a lot like animals? Come to think of it, they (and we) *are* animals. Similar principles and methods work with each, and I had my run at both—dog and (maybe) cat trainer, and kid dad and trainer. We've learned much from both in our history of experimental psychology and behavior analysis.

At the risk of confirming the accusation we psychologists, and men in general, have learned to treat our wives and girlfriends (among others) using the same methods we employ to train (I mean, lovingly guide) our animals—there are some stories I'd like to share about some special animals—and how they affected our fields of psychology, and especially me and my learning and development as a future psychologist. In a real way, my transition from child to adult psychology was mediated in and through dog training and cat craziness. What? I'll explain.

I was a pretty good trainer of my three dogs and then my service dog, Barnabas (he wasn't *just* a dog, mind you)—though not so much the cats. I'll get to those stories, but first I should start with psychology and its famed animal experiments and experimenters.

Animal Psychology

Pavlov's Cats
You probably have heard about Pavlov's dogs—the big-tongued droolers who were subjects in his legendary experiment showing that

dogs could be conditioned to salivate when subjected to repeated trials of a stimulus (bell) paired with food powder injected into their mouths. But did you know that Pavlov, our eminent Russian physiologist of psychology lore, was a *cat person* and not a dog person? I bet you didn't. In fact, he didn't like dogs, and as I understand it, they didn't much take to him. So, quite naturally, he turned originally to his beloved cats for this legendary experiment on what we now call classical Pavlovian conditioning.

But this is where it all went wrong, and I venture you know where this is heading. The cats—unlike in the Thorndike experiments demonstrating the reinforcement law of effect—didn't behave. At all. They just looked at him, and then smartly ran away when Pavlov tried to fit them with the nasty food powder insertion device. But the dogs were okay with it.

Disconsolate, Pavlov decided maybe dogs would sit still and let him do the experiment, and there is the rest of the story—like those great animal "experiments" so delightfully illustrated by my favorite cartoonist Gary Larson. In Pavlov's case, only a few of us (including myself and Mr. Larson) know the real story.

You see, I was an "animal psychologist" long before I was a minimally educated and licensed psychologist: I trained dogs and (less so) cats in my parents' family, and then on my own. That qualified me, before I knew about Pavlov, Thorndike, or Skinner—giants in the field of animal behavior experiments from psychology past—not to mention a more recent helpless dog experimenter giant, Martin Seligman.

Now old B.F.—Skinner, that is—liked to have fun and occasionally abuse birds (this was long before Alfred Hitchcock's terrifying movie *The Birds* scared us all away from feathery pecking ones). Strangely, B.F. found that his pigeon subjects had all gone crazy one weekend when they were being automatically reinforced for pecking at a key in their cage, in return, no doubt, for a pellet of food. Come Monday morning, they were acting in bizarre ways—they had gone insane (if birds can actually)—some walking around in circles, some walking with their head under their feet, others holding a wing up and twirling in a circle, and so on, in repetitive crazy fashion. But rather than sending the pigeons back to the supplier with a stern rebuke about sending him those clearly defective fowl, he wanted to find out why they were behaving this way. He kept them alive to study what in the world happened.

Lo and behold, investigating his food-pellet-delivery mechanism, he discovered that the intended variable ratio schedule of reinforcement (food pellet provided at a varying number of key pecks) turned out to be a variable *time* schedule of reinforcement (every so often the food pellet would be delivered, independently of whether or not the bird had pecked the target). Whatever behavior the pigeons were randomly engaging in at the time the food pellet was delivered was reinforced and likely repeated, sometimes with additional peripheral behaviors added to it. Result: bizarre, insane pigeons.

Superstition
He called what happened accidental conditioning, or "superstitious" behavior (borrowing a term previously coined by another). Are you superstitious like that? Don't lie, I know you are. Here's an example from crazy sports guy behavior: I remember the great baseball player and hitting champion, Wade Boggs of the Boston Red Sox, who always had to eat chicken on days of games, believing it helped him to hit. I think we pretty much know that chicken has nothing to do with hitting a baseball (though the "Famous Chicken" mascot formerly of the San Diego Padres might disagree).

According to the story, Wade was apparently in a pretty bad hitting slump when one day before the game he had chicken, and then went four-for-four hitting. The next day he had chicken, and on it went along with his hitting streak. You get the idea. We all are guilty of superstitious behavior like this—we don't have to be a sports star or fan—just like those pigeons who, behaving in a certain way when the food pellet rolled down the delivery tube, kept doing it until another was delivered, and so on. Am I right? Of course, I am.

A final dog-hating research psychologist I want to uncover is Dr. Marty Seligman. Okay, maybe he didn't hate dogs—probably had one or more at home like the rest of us. But you would think he hated them nonetheless by the way he experimented on them. Granted, the experiment was a very important one, and led to the concept of "learned helplessness" and his later seminal work on optimism, both learned and applied. Nevertheless, Seligman might have gone down the road Pavlov took with cats, but I rather doubt it—especially for an experiment such as Marty's in which he shocked the crap out of those helpless canine experimental subjects. But it was research, so it was okay. The cats, not okay with it—would not even enter the laboratory once they smelled the ruse.

But the dutiful, trusting dogs did, even tolerating the harness they were strapped to, and not realizing the funny "grid" they were standing on was an electrified shock device. Seligman paired a bell sound with unavoidable shock (!) instead of injecting yummy food powder like Pavlov did—to condition an aversive response in his less fortunate dogs. Bell rings, shock administered, dogs freak, but can't escape because of the harness holding them, and so after a series of trials, just stood and took it. Actually, they did whimper, cry, and pee all over the experimental enclosure. A classic fear and terror response. Now guess what happened when he took the harness off. Did you? The dogs did not jump out or run away, even though they could. They felt helpless and acted as such. The "control" group dogs, that had never been harnessed, learned quickly to jump and get the heck out of Dodge.

Seligman had shown what he termed "learned helplessness," which illustrated what can happen with people subjected to aversive, even terrorizing or painful stimuli they could not escape—phobic anxiety and maybe paralyzing PTSD—when near or around those places and memory triggers similar to the terrorizing event. Seligman, also a renowned depression researcher (and then "father" of the new field of positive psychology), compared this phenomenon to people who are depressed, in that they have learned to be helpless over their circumstances, emotions, and depression in similar ways—but could learn and function as an optimistic person—the opposite of a depressed and helpless person. I'm thinking the dogs could be and were as well, though it's hard to imagine a depressed dog other than one who has been abused or traumatized over a period of years, as some rescued dogs are.

Let me turn now a bit away from the psychology history of animal experiments to the family venue. You know, those pet companions from whom we learned so much psychology.

Reigning Cats and Dogs—The Home Menagerie

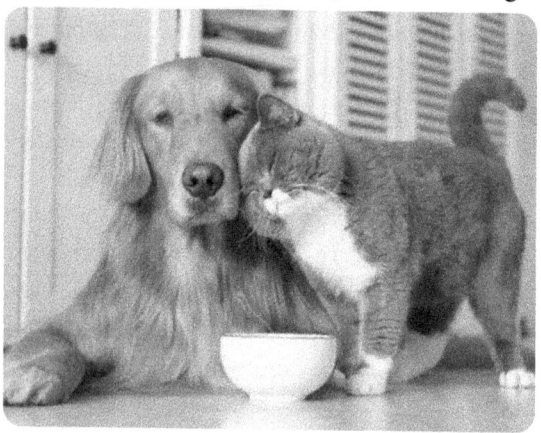

Not to slight the lovely cat people, but I'll start with my dog psychology stories. They stay still more and can be trained, unlike those stupid cats. I didn't really mean that. Cats are smart, too smart for my own good, and usually for any sensible animal psychology experiments. Nevertheless, I've had some very cool cats to tell you about as well, so you strange cat people hang on.

Bruno

The first animal our family had that I remember as a little boy was a big brown standard poodle named Bruno. It was a good name for him

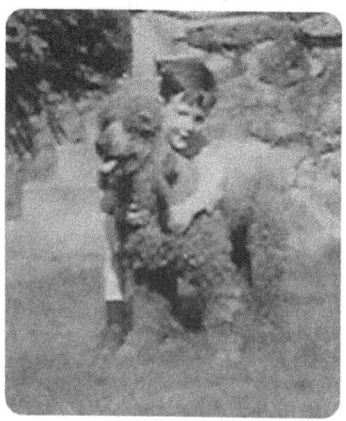

because he had a guy's personality, I believe. Now poodles are kind of a strange breed, but this particular poodle was not one of those you give that froufrou stupid cut with the puffy tail and legs, and the bouffant head cut that makes them look silly and girly. Bruno was *all guy*. He was left to be a dog, uncut (no, not that, I mean his fur) and unabused by girly groomers.

Animal Psychology

I think back with pride on how Bruno once tried to jump through a screen door at a delivery man he decided was a threat to our family—or just thought it would be fun to scare the crap out of that guy, and he did. By the way, mail carriers ceased to come to our door after that (we were allowed to come get our mail at the back door to the local post office, left in a pile with our name taped to the top for the next several years, that is until the old mailman had died and the rest forgot about the incident). Dog family penance.

Bruno was also a confident man-dog who liked to lie in the street, an important part of his territory to occupy and protect—like humans will do (back when dogs could roam free in a neighborhood and make their way back to home for feeding times).

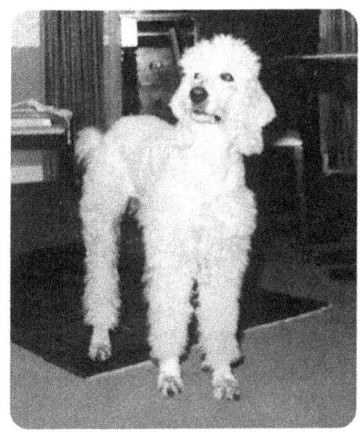

Nipper

After Bruno there was Nipper, a white male poodle who, for some unfathomable reason, my father and mother decided to make into a girly girl with a froufrou haircut. Oh, all right, you poodle lovers. They could be nice dogs, and smart, and we loved our Bruno. What we humans do to abuse our animals, akin to how we alter who our kids are meant to be and live—the old "spittin'" image, "you will become exactly like me" manipulation. Or to make them the opposite, humiliating them before all to see. Like Nipper. Poor dog.

For example, we would race through the house, with him in joyful pursuit, run down the carpeted stairs to the lower slickly tiled floor. When he hit the floor at full speed, his feet would fly out from under him, splaying like a cartoon character, invoking the nails out protective instinct, and he would slide all the more dangerously onto his side or back and slam into the wall! We thought that was the funniest thing we had ever seen. So we'd do it again and again with this loving, not-so-smart creature, a willing participant each time. I'm thinking that was kid-to-dog abuse. But there was more…

151

Not satisfied, we would play this "game" with him in which we would call his name over and over again, with him right in front of us, and pretend not to see him. We could do that for hours. It drove him crazy. We loved it. I think he defined insanity for us at an early age: doing the same thing over and over again and expecting different results. It was a Charlie Brown and Lucy football-holding moment that we, as Lucy, kept pulling on poor Nipper. Kids can be so mean—animal-to-animal abuse. Should have been illegal (might be now).

Duke

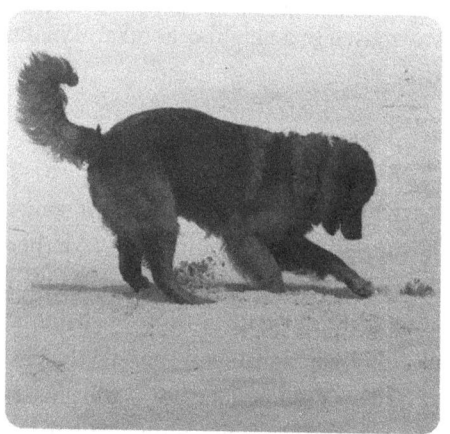

When I became of age to have a dog, I got a great golden retriever who loved to swim for hours at a time in my parents' backyard pool, when he wasn't digging like mad at the beach for crabs like this. And Duke was a great swimmer, as all retrievers are with their webbed feet and powerful rudder-like tail. He would swim slowly around in easy circles, with just the top of his head and eyes above water, and tail steering, like a gator. But we learned when he was in the pool, no one else would dare try to swim there. He seemed to have the notion that it was his *job* to "save" anyone who got in the pool to swim and therefore would swim furiously over to whatever body was trying to float or swim there, *and get up on top of them.* He didn't quite get the concept of saving.

I also honed my behavior modification techniques with Duke. It was too late for the poodles, and I was too young to master the techniques—not that they would have worked on the poodles (Bruno needed no training at all). I taught Duke to balance a dog biscuit on his broad retriever nose, waiting for the "okay" to flip it up in the air and catch it (if it hit the ground, it was mine). I think this is a required part of training for goldens and Labs, and, of course, it was a great party trick. Naturally, I taught my two Labs after Duke to do that as well.

But for Duke, I could leave a whole steak on a plate on the floor, put him in stay position in front of it, walk out the door, drive away, and come back 10 minutes later, and the steak was still there, untouched. I wouldn't give him the steak. I was such a mean trainer. But he loved me. I dare you to try that with your dog (or cat!) *or kid*. Forget it. I also taught him to say "yum" to get an ice cube. I was the best dog trainer I knew. When it came to people, I didn't always do so well. You've figured that already, though.

I once applied my behavior modification dog "expertise" when Duke ran across a broken bottle and severed his wrist almost completely during a run with me. I rushed him to the university vet school ER (where I knew poor graduate students could get free care if they could use the animal for training purposes). They operated on him overnight and called me a day later. He had chewed off three casts and they weren't sure how to stop him from tearing the stitches and causing loss of the foot. B Mod guy to the rescue: I had them release him to me, with heavily taped-up leg and foot, and I instituted the Tabasco aversive conditioning intervention. Each trial included my waiting with Tabasco bottle in hand and squirting a liberal amount of the Tabasco hot sauce into his mouth (poor dog, evil master—but I was *saving* his foot!) each time he went to bite off the tape, combined with a shout, "NO!" Many trials later—success! Sort of. He stopped trying to tear the tape off, eventually, and the wrist and foot went on to heal completely. But he required Tabasco on his food from then on.

Following my "brilliant" attempt as an animal behaviorist, veterinarian "consultant," I used a principle of discipline with my dog Duke, and then all the rest. Not too many people understand that when it comes to their dogs—not to mention kids, spouses, or others that you like—*never* call them to punish them (you've heard it: "honey, we need to talk"). When they come to you, it should always result in a reward or positive thing—like a pet, a scratch behind the ear (only for animals), and a kind word, kiss, or hug (humans. Okay, dogs, too). If they need to be disciplined (corrected or confronted), then go to them (if you can catch them). Duke understood this principle well. When he knew he was in trouble over some infraction, and I was approaching him with a harsh word and possibly a rolled newspaper in my hand for gentle but firm swat purposes, he would turn, not to run away *from* me, but *toward* me. He knew. Smart dog.

Isaac, the Character

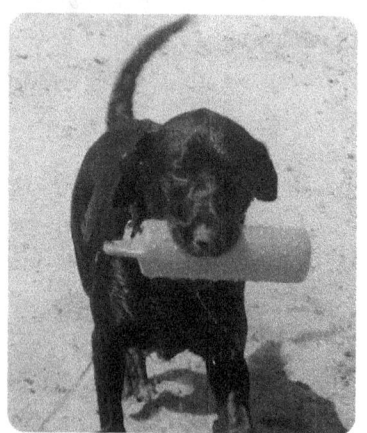

Isaac was my first Lab, after two goldens, and he was a big, black, smart, and canny one. We named him Isaac because in Hebrew it means "laughter," and he definitely made us laugh as he expressed his great personality. It was a different kind of dog psychology for us—crazy humor with gentle love, along with an irritating independent streak. When he was in trouble for chewing something he shouldn't have, I would put him in timeout in the corner of the room. But he knew, it seemed, that if he could break us up in laughter, he could be forgiven and released from his purgatory to rejoin the family. He would roll over on his back and look at us upside down with this big grin of white teeth at us. How could we *not* laugh? Reprieve!

Isaac loved to swim and retrieve. DUH, he's a LAB! Throw anything, I mean anything, into the water, and he was *in*. It was his *duty*. Getting the throw buoy like you see in the picture was nothing. One time he pulled in a whole huge pine tree, dragging it out of the lake by its very tip. Wow. I would sometimes have some fun throwing multiple buoys in, one after the other, as he was bringing the one in. He'd just drop that one, go out and corral the others and eventually get them all up to the shore, for great celebratory praise from me! He would do anything, it seemed, for that praise; but that occasional yum-yum treat was appreciated too.

As all swimming expert retrievers, Isaac especially loved to go to the beach. He'd start smelling the ocean at about the one-mile mark

Animal Psychology

and get all excited, whining and pacing in the car. I'm like that when I, too, get a whiff of those cinnamon buns at the mall, possibly without the whining and pacing. What we didn't know until a surfer brought him to us, was that he loved to surf. He would swim out through the waves at the dog beach, out to where the surfers were sitting on their boards, and get up on the nearest surfboard—whether or not he was invited! "Is this your crazy dog?" they'd confront us. "Nope, never seen him," would be our reply. Crazy dog.

But Isaac was loved. Here he is with his "boy" Josh, chewing his big bone and being "serenaded." I'm not sure what the T-shirt was about. Probably something put on by his musician, co-troublemaker, just for fun. And he put up with it, of course.

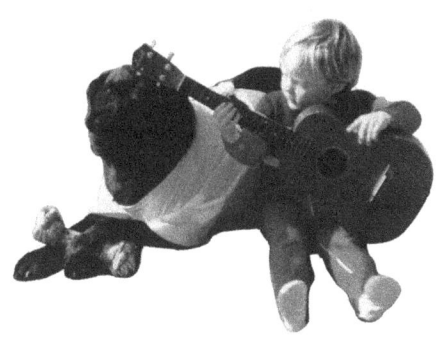

We never fixed Isaac (how could we!), if you know what I mean (of course you do), and so he was a wanderer, always looking for ladies, and sometimes pie. We'd regularly get a call from a local pie shop in town after one of his escapes. "Isaac's here," the caller said from town. "He's fine, just getting some [actual] pie from the customers. We'll send him home soon, or you can come get him." My wife kept seeing little puppies around town in yards that looked an awful lot like Isaac.

Isaac's combination of people loving, wanderlust carousing, pie begging escapee-joyfulness sometimes got him in trouble. He was one of those special breeds who could grin. Really. Have you seen them? I had a friend with a Dalmatian who did it too. When Isaac was happy to see you, and maybe a bit embarrassed, he would show his teeth in a funny, toothy grin at people. If you didn't know him, you might think he was about to bite you. But, no, he was happy to see you, grinningly. Yet not everyone knew that and so were not as equally happy to see those big dog teeth displays. One day, the local sheriff called us saying someone had complained that our dog was threatening to bite them, and he was required to call animal control about our vicious, threatening animal. I think our laughing at the situation, once we figured what had happened, didn't help calm the sheriff, and our attempt at explanation didn't go so far either, but we were able to retrieve our goofy retriever, silly grinner, and most appropriately named boy.

"*Isaac, that's not a cat!*" his mommy yelled from the porch as he broke through the doorway one night after that white-striped "cat." Need I say more? I won't. He caught it, of course, and nights and days of tomato juice baths later… Bad dog.

Nevertheless, Isaac loved chasing cats, though no longer interested in those with the white stripes (we call that "one trial learning") and seemed especially delighted in those furry fun runs. What could be better! Now what to do if he *ever* caught one is a different "good question" that frankly doesn't need answering, since fortunately he never did. But his cat-chasing instinct seems to be what we also call in psych lingo a natural reinforcer, which means in a free operant (uncontrolled) setting the behavior will occur on its own, no matter what. We sometimes will discover reinforcers for kids and people by just watching them. What they tend to do is the thing they like to do. The so-called grandmother's rule, we call contingency management, is to allow the person or animal to do what they love to do only *after* the required behavior. "Do this, and *then* you get the cookie" (or sex) (sorry about that). Some get this process wrong. They give the reinforcer of the behavior or reward *before* the behavior. This is called a bribe and doesn't really work. Definitely not with dogs.

Anyway, Isaac the Lab grew up with a couple cats in our homes, and so was well versed in their wily ways, but often not quite as smart or quick (or evil) as they were. One of our cats, who trained him through his puppyhood, would bring in birds from outdoors and set them free for the fun of it (probably to eventually eat them after another fun indoors "hunt"). Isaac would then find the bird, maybe partly disabled by the cat, take them in his soft mouth, and let them go outside. Good dog!

It was a game they both seemed to enjoy, but the cat was sometimes not done before creating a new game. We also kept finding Isaac locked in the small second bathroom when we would come home from an outing. We couldn't for the life of us figure out how he got in there, as we would hear his whimpering from behind the door. Finally figuring it out, we imagined the cat batting him on the head as he rounded the corner by the couch, then racing with Isaac in hot pursuit to the bathroom, going in between the door and the wall, and slipping out as Isaac pushed his way into the space between, closing the door! Bad cat!

Barnabas (Velo)

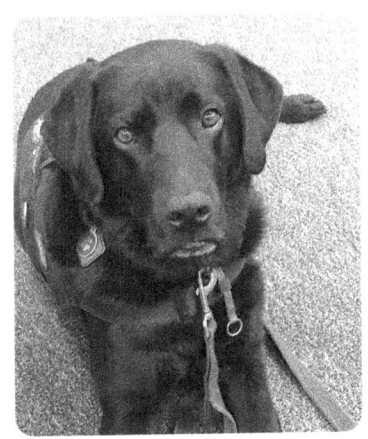

My most recent dog was a wonderful service dog named Velo. I renamed him Barnabas for the biblical meaning of the name, "son of encouragement." He was a great encouragement and encourager to me during some of my recovery time from PTSD, and in my work with veterans with PTSD (which you will read about soon) as a part of my clinical practice.

Barnabas, or Velo, was a purebred black Labrador retriever, bred by the Guide Dogs of America program of Southern California (GDA is a great organization to give donations to). I was on the waiting list for a large male through the program for service dogs for first responders and military vets (called Next Step Service Dogs, NSSD, of Escondido, CA, another great program that does so much good, so consider a donation to them if you might). Then he was returned to GDA because the blind woman got sick and could not use him, so GDA offered him to NSSD (and me!). I was told when I went to decide whether to take him that I would have just a few minutes to decide. We both enthusiastically decided almost immediately with licks, pats, and rapid "show-off" compliance with a few basic commands of "sit," "down," and "paw." "I'll take him!"

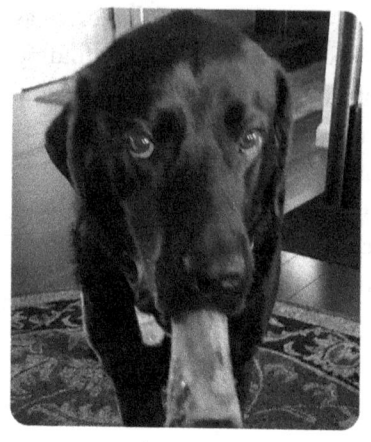

No, Barnabas in the picture here is not smoking a bong (dogs don't need chilling out—they already *are* chill, especially Labs!), though it looks a lot like that. It was one of his favorite bones, marrow extracted already, but tasty enough. No one taught him how to carry it. He had his own style, and I think he was proudly showing it off to me as I took the picture.

He's now nine years old (he was 2 1/2 then) and has become a family member in our home. Actually, he loves my wife, his "mommy," more than me as she walks him more, brushes him, and sings to him at night—even though I'm his "master" and am the only one to feed him. Love conquers duty and stomach apparently, once again.

This big black service dog was bred, selected, and trained as a guide dog for the blind and then for first responders and veterans with PTSD in one most special way—to avoid risky places and people—in order to protect his handler companion. I wouldn't have imagined it possible, but sometimes he would alert me to a potential "danger" with his ears, look at the "threat" and then at me, and sometimes try to lead me in the opposite direction, kind of like that lane assist steering wheel nudge in our newer bells and whistles–equipped cars. One time, we were working with a huge ex-Marine with some pretty major PTSD and scary anger, and Barnabas would not even come close to say hello or camp at the feet of this veteran client as he usually did. He went to the farthest place in the office and stayed there the whole session until he left. I even called him over to greet the man, but he would not.

This sensitivity to threat avoidance applied to me as well. When I once inquired of our trainers at NSSD how he could be trained to interrupt and calm me when I became triggered or upset, they asked what he did when that happened. I explained that when I was reacting with anger and usually loud voice to some sudden (frightening) sound or unwanted surprise, for example when touched from behind by someone, he would get up from beside me and walk off, fearfully. "Then what did you do?" I was asked. I would immediately notice his fearful departure, lower my voice, sweetly and calmly call him back, and lovingly pet him. "So there you go," was their response. I got it.

Surprisingly, though perhaps similarly, he seems to be frightened of guns. A hunting dog like a Lab? Really. Well, at least at the loud sounds they can make. I don't think he has ever heard an actual gunshot, but I once was cleaning a couple rifles in my home and when I cocked it for cleaning purposes, he quickly retreated to the farthest reaches of our house—back where he goes during thunderstorms, Fourth of July, and Blue Angels air shows. The noise frightened him, and maybe something about the violence and threat of a gun. Maybe not. But several days later, he saw me taking one rifle out of the case and he pushed his way behind my wife for protection. He's never done that. The next day when we brought two rifles out of the car to go to the shooting range, he wouldn't come out of the building and hid behind their bathroom door! Wow. He somehow detected danger or threat and signaled me to that fact with his rare and strategic avoidance behavior. Our PTSD dog trainers and the GDA would be proud. I must tell them about that.

Not surprising, Barnabas's gentle personality was exceptionally polite as well. In the mornings, he will not bother me (but he will my wife, his mommy) before I am ready to get up. He will raise his head up to catch my eye, and if I'm just rolling over and not looking at him, will put it back down and try to get to sleep once again. I wish we could train our kids, and maybe irritating spouses, to do that—but I guess it must be genetic, so forget it. When I reach for him or call to come, he comes with a powerful wagging tail (their tails are known to be coffee table sweepers, registered weapons) and greeting "huffs" and "down dog" yoga bows—our grand time of good morning happy hello. (He is a pro at the yoga classes I sometimes take him to, imitating all our dog-like positions.)

Then comes eating time, Barnabas's favorite. Need I tell you he is a voracious eater? Labs eat *fast*, wolfing the food down with nary a graze over a single taste bud, possibly upsetting their stomachs, that a special bowl had to be invented. It's a cool creation. It has ridges and mountains and valleys in it, in an attempt to slow them down. Hardly. But nice try; remember that massive tongue. To add to his feeding frustration, I also make him (maybe "make" is not the most spiritual word here)—invite him—to pray before he can eat. I use the Chinese word for "pray"—which sounds a lot like "dow gaugh" the way I badly pronounce it—and he goes immediately to his down position, lying out, crossing his paws in an attempt to be sufficiently holy or worthy, I'm guessing, until he gets the "...*in Jesus's name*! EAT." I tried to train him to lower his head during this "prayer time," but that was just too much for him (as well as the Pavlovian drool puddle on the floor by then), so I gave it up.

Sometimes when we are in church and he hears that wonderful phrase, his ears perk up and uncontrollable salivation begins (Pavlov would be proud). (He *is* a service dog, so he gets to go pretty much everywhere with me, special vest and all). Sometimes I am in a different room when he rushes back in from his mommy-walk, making a beeline to the bowl, when he finds it full but no "daddy" there for the obligatory prayer. So, he waits, standing there, eyes on the bowl, ears tuned into the sound of my steps. He won't eat until he prays and is given the command to "eat." Sometimes it's five minutes or more when I'm off doing something else and forget, and then I find him there frozen by the bowl position. He still won't eat until the prayer. Amazing dog. Maybe people should be more like that. I think I've established this already. If not, read on.

For exercise, I got a great dog leash bike attachment and would take him out for brief exercise bouts, but he never liked that, and his pads could burn on the asphalt during the day if I was not careful to test the pavement before starting (if you can't hold your hand down for six seconds without burning them, it's too hot for their feet and pads). As a result, I decided to try a different form of exercise that required hardly any effort from me: the treadmill. Let's just say he wants *nothing* to do with this crazy earthquaking contraption with the floating "sidewalk." My training with hamburger meat has only gotten him to stand there for some seconds and take a few steps.

He was just too smart for my unsophisticated and faulty attempts to get him to do things that were not a part of his service training or mentality. By the way, did I tell you he knows how to use mirrors to look at you? He does. I catch him all the time looking at me in the mirror to save him the "trouble" of lifting and turning his huge head when I'm speaking to him or he is giving me the shame stare of a "starving dog" needing food! I've never had or heard of a dog who did that.

Barnabas, in my mind, is a nearly perfect service animal, in which most all the Labrador-dogginess was bred out to enhance his service training and traits. He wasn't interested in birds or ducks, tennis balls or retrieving anything. Amazing. It was like he just wanted to serve. Oh, okay, eating and sleeping, smelling and peeing too. Swimming? Not hardly. He would wade into the ocean up to about his ankles and didn't like the waves there at the Southern California dog beaches I would take him to.

But now we have just entered him in swim therapy at a great program near us in Costa Mesa, CA (Animal Wellness Center), and he just had his second "lesson" in the pool there. Can you imagine a nine-year-old Lab who has never swam? Believe it. His first couple entrances into the water off the doggie platform require two very strong female trainers trying to lift him, nails out gripping the wooden platform for life, into the water. It was cool watching him figure out what those webbed feet were for and what those powerful arms and legs were designed to do in the water. He's now a champion swimmer, though with some human help (he's just shed the doggie life vest). Way to go big boy! Mom and Dad were so proud of him.

We are still working on getting his 120-plus pounds down to his goal weight (I should say my goal weight for him, not his goal) of 95 pounds. I'm losing the battle, but the swim therapy to the rescue. He's a big dog and wants to be bigger! When occasionally "corrected" by do-gooding friends who comment on how overweight he is (i.e., you owners should be ashamed for letting him become like that!), I have learned to ask them if they have ever seen an older Lab who was skinny. Enuf said.

But, he's loved a lot, probably too much, and how many dogs do you know (we ask him) that have five dog beds and a mommy who sings to him almost every night? "That's right, and don't you forget it!" I'll tell you some more about this special creature when I discuss PTSD, his second training with me. But a little more on dog therapy if you will humor me.

Dog Therapy

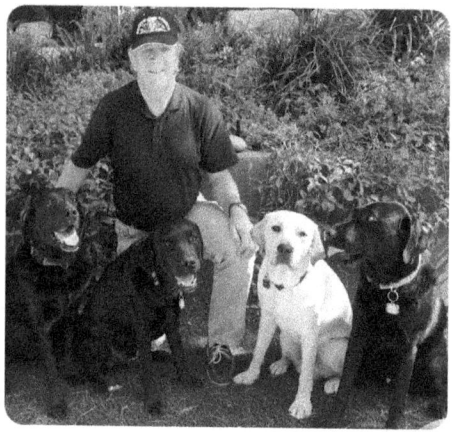

I had a good friend and fraternity brother from college (Billy H.) who, along with my bio teaching helper (Kerry from an earlier story), followed me down to my university master's program in psychology and started with me in the educational psychology program I told you about earlier. Bill was a golden retriever lover like myself, though I graduated to the Labrador retriever afterwards. (Some would say it was a step down, but not me.)

Bill did a brilliant thing with his dog as a class assignment. He brought his sweet, happy, loving golden to class in order to demonstrate to the class a type of counseling approach. On his day to make his presentation, Bill brought the dog in, sat down, and without a word let him hustle around, tail wagging furiously, happy face (you know dogs can have happy faces, don't you?), and greeting every person in the small circle of classmates. It enlivened the class with love and happiness, that not a word was needed. It was the example of client-centered counseling and therapy—pure empathy and unconditional love. I'm certain Bill got an "A" on the assignment. I loved it, and I think Carl Rogers would have too.

I once had a client, years later, who was a high-stress, self-absorbed man who struggled with anger and relationship breakdowns—and he didn't much care for dogs, especially not mine. As a Type A person (he called himself a Type A+++), he tended to care little for those things, people or pets that could do little for him, and a dog was no different. When I brought my service dog Barnabas into the therapy room, he was both disinterested and partially unhappy with having a dog there to take focus off him. I could tell by his standoffishness and facial expression of apparent dislike. No worries, but I was curious.

Even so, the lovingness of Barnabas broke through his wall so that by about the third session they were great friends. Okay, not great friends, but tolerant ones. Not long after, he thought about 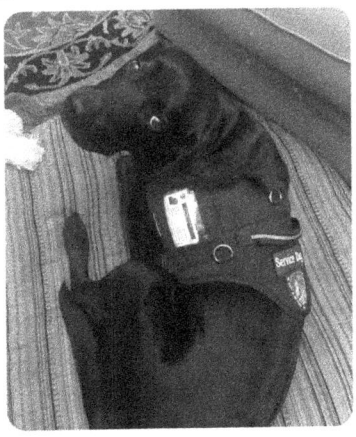 the possibility of getting a service dog for his diabetes—a "sugar sniffer." He eventually applied and got one for himself—a beautiful labradoodle he named "Shoogie" (get it?) (I take back everything bad I said about poodles) who trained together with him to alert him when his blood sugar levels were off—one time even saving his life when he was in trouble and near coma.

Cat-ology

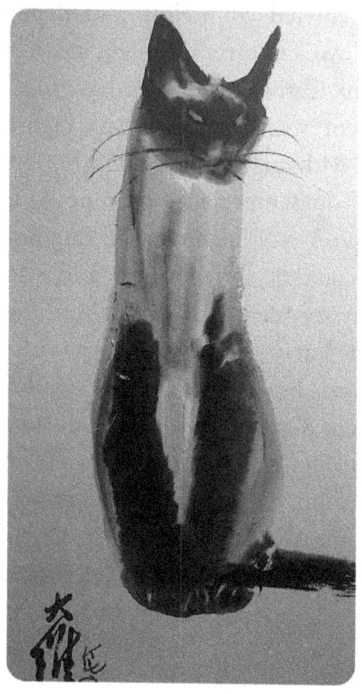

"Dogs come when they're called; cats take a message and get back to you."

—MISSY DIZICK

Siamese Training

My family growing up was a dog *and* cat family. It was one of those saving graces that gave love, humor, and a semblance of normalcy to us weird kids. My parents were originally cat people, having two Siamese cats during their time in New York City. My dad trained them to use the toilet. I never witnessed this miraculous feat but trusted that we were not being lied to. Mostly this was before us kids, but I do remember one cat who came later, a big blue point who used the doorstopper spring to pull out and snap when he wanted back in. Dad told me it was his doorbell. I didn't argue that night when the sound scared me and Dad leaned over and opened the kitchen door, letting him saunter through, looking of course for his special meal of chicken livers and steak pieces (Dad spoiled them. Need I say that?).

Animal Psychology

Gandalf

The next cat after the smart tabby that "trained" and had cat-fun with Isaac was my favorite, a longhaired Manx cat—the kind with no tail (a nub). He looked like a wildcat or lynx. He had six toes with a big frock of gray-and-white hair. His look reminded me of Gandalf from the *Lord of the Rings*, so the name stuck. He was the most interesting animal. I got him as a tiny kitten from my pastor's ranch home at one Christmas party when I commented to him about what a cool cat he was. "You want him?" he asked. The rest was history.

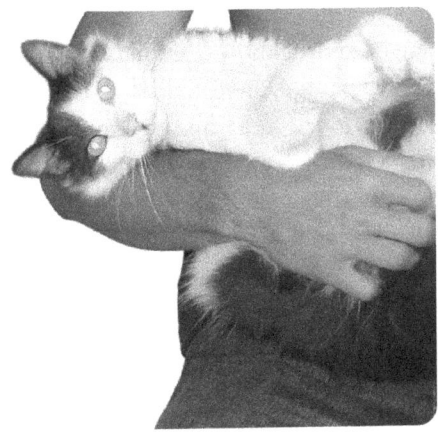

Gandalf came to live with me on my old beat-up 46-foot ketch I sailed down from LA to San Diego and lived on for a few years after my divorce. I figured, if I couldn't have a wife and family home, I could get a lifelong fantasy of a sailboat and live on it. Bachelor's dream! Not exactly. One mooring (a buoy anchored to the sea bottom with a float ball for boat hookups) I had it on was under the Coronado Bridge, just off the shore of ritzy Coronado Island. I would tell friends who asked where I was living that I was at Coronado, on the water, with a 360-degree view of the ocean—not bothering to reveal it was on an old leaky boat riding the tide. They figured I must have been very rich, though some knew better than to ask.

One day, Gandalf trained *me* to play fetch. You see, I had thoughtlessly crumpled up a piece of paper and threw it across the cabin from my bunk. Next thing I knew Gandalf jumped down, picked it up in his teeth, and brought it back to me. When I saw what he had done—fetch like a dog—I decided to reward him each time he did it. He seemed to like doing it, and we had a lot of fun with that game. Then came the demonstration for my friends and family.

"Watch what Gandalf can do!" With rapt attention, they would watch me crumple up the paper and throw it across the room, and I'd say, "Gandalf, fetch!" He'd just look at me, as if to say, "naa, I don't feel like it." Darn cat. Another Lucy and Charlie Brown football pull.

I remember when Gandalf decided to try to eat a duck. He had never had one, and I'm not sure he even knew what they were. They would swim up to our boat, with Gandalf now leaning way over watching with rapt attention, probably thinking, "that creature looks like it would be good to catch and eat" (in cat language, of course). Next thing I know, I hear a splash, and Gandalf has jumped on top of a suspecting duck. But what he didn't know was that ducks can dive and swim, neither of which he could or would do. I think he danced across the water to get back to the boat, and never tried that feat again.

What Gandalf also dreamed of trying was capturing and eating birds, no matter how big, on land of course. We were tied up at the public dock one day and there was a very big blue heron standing there. It towered over Gandalf, but no matter. Gandalf tried to make a "stealth" attempt on the heron. Needless to say, the heron saw him and was not too concerned. A couple sailors and I watched this scene.

Finally, close enough to make his final attack, Gandalf rushed at the big bird, who calmly flapped his wings a couple times, enough to rise above the attacking stupid cat, peck him on the head, and then settle back down, not losing an inch of ground. Gandalf ran off, ego hurting but still alive. Phew. He never tried that land-bird attack in the future. When I sold the boat and moved to another city, I gave him to my ex who lived in the mountains, where he lived out his life hunting various things, until one day he just apparently disappeared. He was a great cat and turned this dog guy into a dog and cat person in a wonderful way.

Bubba and Rocky
Is it possible for a cat to be more like a dog? Absolutely. Gandalf certainly was, and then there are my brother's two cat-dogs, Bubba and Rocky. Here they are with their human servant, my brother, David. They are known as Maine coons and have those unique

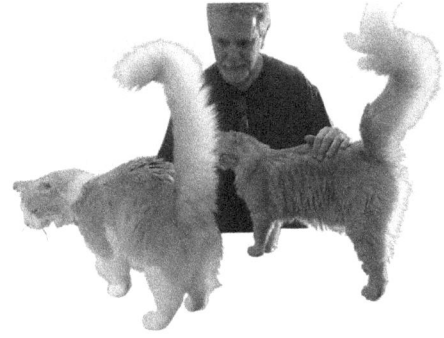

characteristics that bridge the gap between monkeys, cats and dogs. I guess that's why my brother and I—dog people—like them so much. Would you believe these very large, wild-looking cats—with huge, fluffy but monkey-like and probably tree branch–gripping prehensile tails that can lay all the way across their backs and heads—actually growl and bark! Like *dogs!* When a stranger like me comes to the door, they go into protective and (God forbid) attack mode. They are also affectionate in a dog kind of way. What's strangest of all, though, is that they *wag their tails like dogs when they are excitedly happy.* Say what?

Talk about a strange animal psychology! When they are most joyful and happy, the tail vibrates. Are you kidding? Nope. I've seen it. Any other cat that "wags" its tail is *not* happy. Get ready for attack. Not these two. Get ready for loving purrs, head rubs, and dog-like lying down for belly rubs. Some say we humans used to have tails. Imagine trying to figure out what the tail wag means—love or attack. I think our facial expressions serve the tail function in us humans, don't you?

Indeed, the animal world of cat and dog behavior tells us a lot about ourselves, and it's why we observe them intently and even experiment on them. They are curious creatures worthy of our love and attention. But there are a couple of other animals I believe should be especially voted into our psychological menagerie Hall of Fame—monkeys (who are a lot like us, we know), and bears and horses (who are not). The contrast of those tree-swinging, honey-and-grub-slurping, and landbound hoofers is interestingly different from the dog and cat classroom we are just leaving, and they have held a place of honor in the world of animal psychology. For example...

Monkey Business

After an awful experience freezing at my child psych lecture as a graduate teaching assistant—that was no lecture at all—I seemed unable to get out of psychology despite my great efforts. So, I eventually transferred to another professor. This new professor was a physiological psychologist, an area much more interesting to me than the decision factors of the old prof. The new one was doing research with, of all things, chimps, and controlling them with brain electrode implantation into their emotional and other centers. Now, I know that chimps are not exactly monkeys, so allow me the sweeping overgeneralization that they look similar to monkeys, so monkeys they will be for our purposes—noting I am the storyteller and author of this animal *hazarai* after all.

The research was conducted in part at the largest chimp colony in the US, where the government also did some early rocket and space research using the chimps to test for effects on them of g-forces with rocket sleds, and survival and physical reactions to rocket and space flight. It was only an hour's drive from my university. I'll never forget my first visit to that facility. Walking through the center, with all the chimps in cages, many of them huge, I noticed some of the handlers had fingers missing on their hands. Can you guess why? Come to find out if they got too close to the older chimps (teenage and up), the chimps would grab the arm or hand of the one too close and bite the fingers off!

My professor told me about the time he accidentally got too close to one of the chimp enclosures and his arm was grabbed by an adult chimp. A chimp's or ape's strength is approximately six-to-one of a male human—a 100-pound chimpanzee is as strong and powerful as a 600-pound muscular man. Woah! So, when the professor was in the grip of the chimp, who could easily pull his arm completely off, all he could do was freeze (fight-or-flight response was not available). Eventually, the chimp let him go, arm sore but intact. I walked a wide path around the enclosures after that!

The Bear Truth

Bears are nothing like us. Their psychology is far from human, or even dog-like, and (important point here) they will *eat you*. Like me and Dad, my mom was an animal lover. But come to find out, she was such a talented and courageous animal trainer (I believe those traits helped her to understand and deal with her brood of five pathological kids) that she even loved to work with dangerous animals. *Like bears!*

Dad told me the story of when they were vacationing up at a mountain cabin and playing bridge with some friends. All of a sudden, outside on the deck in front of the large picture window facing their bridge table, a huge brown bear reared up and filled the whole window, facing them—paws and claws reaching the top. Everyone but Mom freaked out, screaming no doubt, like normal people would. But not Mom, the "abnormal." She calmly said: "Oh, that's just George. He came for his lunch." Mom walked into the kitchen, got him bear food of some sort (could have been just about anything edible, I'm told), and went out on the porch to feed George. BUT THEY LET HER! Nobody was killed, as far as I know, but WHY DIDN'T MY FATHER—LOVING HUSBAND—STOP THIS CRAZY WIFE OF HIS FROM TRYING TO BE EATEN BY A WILD BEAR, AND ALL OF THEM DEVOURED AS WELL WHEN HE WAS STILL HUNGRY? No idea. I guess Dad had learned the psychology of when to try to stop someone intent on even crazy action, and when to not even try. This, I'm guessing, was a "don't even try" occasion, even risking sure mauling and death to all.

Horsing Around

There was a kinder, personal side of my "evil friend," fellow psychology graduate student and helper, Murray (remember the big contract for writing my doctoral thesis?). He was a rancher and horseman from New Mexico and once helped train—desensitize, I should say—my first wife's year-old colt. Anyone who knows anything about year-old colts knows they can be wild. No, they ARE WILD. And Sierra was. Murray showed up at our corral with many very strange objects: umbrellas, noisemakers, lights, and things, and began opening and closing the umbrella, making all kinds of noises, shining lights, etc. The horse, tied to the fence rail, was going crazy. After a while, he calmed down. Desensitization. It worked.

Crazy Horse

Sensitization happened to me in another horse story. When I was at the children's hospital working, one of my friends, an orthopedic surgery resident, was another horseman who had two horses. When he invited me to go for a ride with him, I gladly agreed, which was my first mistake. The second was getting up on the horse he offered me. I think it was the better of the two, not that you would have known it by what happened, and I believe it was a setup.

No sooner had I swung my leg up and settled into the western saddle, this crazy horse began to jump, left and right, forward and back, turning around, and rearing up. Insanity. All the while I was trying to control the horse, my now ex-buddy was rolling on the ground in uproarious laughter (I think his other horse must have been laughing too, but I was too distracted to notice). I finally managed to jump off this mad beast, barely surviving with my life and non-broken back and limbs, and I demanded an explanation. WHAT IS WRONG WITH THIS INSANE HORSE?!

Come to find out the horse was a finely tuned, highly trained, and sensitive horse who had been pressure trained, and every slight pressure I exerted unknowingly with my knees or heels or hands on the reigns was sending a signal to him as to what I wanted him to do. And he kept trying to do it, little doubt wondering to himself, WHAT IS WRONG WITH THIS INSANE *RIDER?* I'VE GOT TO GET HIM OFF ME! He succeeded. It was no contest.

Horse Motivation

Speaking of horses, I learned later in my career about Monty Roberts (even attending one of his wild horse–training demonstrations)—the true *horse whisperer*. His methods and techniques focused on speaking the horse's language (he called it *equus*) and gentling rather than "breaking" them as he trained and motivated the horse to accept a saddle, bridle, and rider. I wondered if my former buddy's crazy horse was touch-trained in this way. Monty's methods have helped transform horse training in a major way, and even the field of motivational counseling of which I later became a student and trainer. I'll say more about this on floor six, so stay tuned.

Animal Personality Disorders

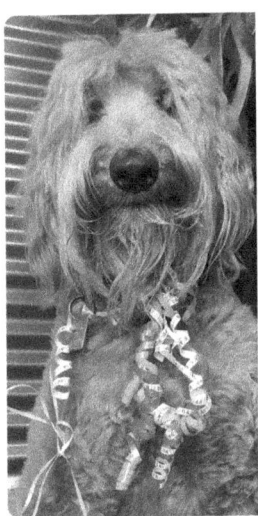
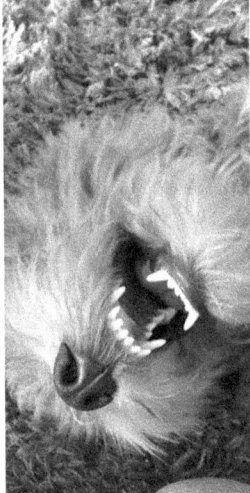
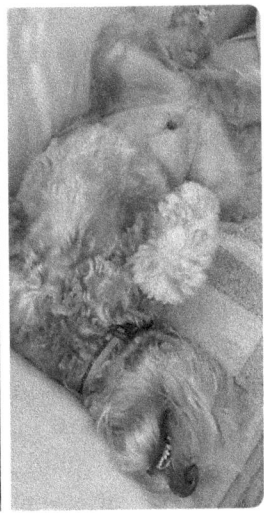

Finally, in concluding our tour through psychology's animal farm and the family petting zoo, have you ever thought that animals could have personality disorders too? Maybe you have one—an animal with a personality disorder, not a personality disorder yourself (though, in truth, they are likely connected). Makes sense they could pick up on and suffer from our own personality disorders, weirdness, and trauma even. Like Willoughby here. He's a nearly perfect example of what facing a three-way, multiple personality/dissociative identity disorder is like, as an Australian/Labrador retriever/poodle mixture, better known as an Aussie-Labradoodle. It's a crazy, confusing intermingling, and Willoughby is that practically pure personification (diagnostically speaking, that is) of a certifiable, but smart, loveable, zany companion. The pictures tell the story.

My father, case in point, had a particular personality that was not only frequently toxic to us kids but also to his stupid poodles. I can't say they became Type A like my dad (you will see later) but they might have, *and* they did have a common form of personality wackiness (partly due to kid-to-poodle trauma-inducing harassment), resulting in a diagnosable condition called "histrionic personality disorder." You can look it up. It's characterized by an insecure self- (or in this case, dog-) centeredness, requiring nearly constant attention and affirmation. You've had dogs like this, yes? Maybe even the little poodles. Perhaps like those hyper highly nervous ones whom the big, *actual* dogs like Bruno, Duke, Isaac, Barnabas, and Willoughby will stop and look so curiously at when confronted by its protectively "vicious" yapping attack, thinking, no doubt, *Are you some kind of a dog, or what?* You know what I'm talking about. I've told you already about those nutty poodles (sorry, once again, you poodle lovers). We all suffered together, and sometimes the loving, even if stupid, dogs were a wonderful saving grace and comfort to and for us, in spite of it all. My service dog for PTSD, Barnabas, served me and my professional clients, and veterans at the VA, in wonderful ways.

Let me now turn to the family psychology stories I've promised. From dogs, cats, monkeys, bears, and horses to humankind. Almost sounds like the evolutionary ladder (excepting bears and horses, of course), but not so much. Anyway, let's jump in and stir up some outlandish, silly, revealing, and sometimes touching family and personal stories as we wind gradually toward the deeper areas of trauma, coping, and recovery.

ROOM 402

CHILD AND FAMILY PSYCHOLOGY

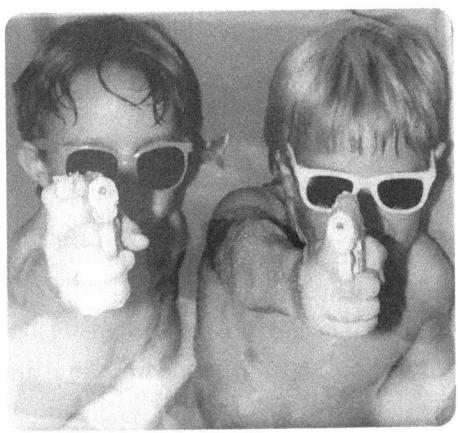

*"Child psychology and child psychiatry cannot be reformed.
They must be abolished."*

—Dr. Thomas Szasz

"All children are essentially criminal."

—Denis Diderot

Much of my learning as a psychologist came from my accidental psychologist-to-be time with kids, especially those in the hospital setting. Of course, we know it's the parents who are the problem, not to mention the child psychologists and psychiatrists who are collecting the rent and pretending to know what to do with them (the kids, that is). I joined the club.

You see, I was a "special ed" teacher, with absolutely *no* education or training in special education. But then, I was special (need I remind you?), and the kids were special, and the teaching was kind of special. Voilà! (And, by the way, nobody asked for my "credentials" or my experience, other than my specialness.) So, there I was. This insidious psychological plot against those poor kids thickened when, by proxy, I became a consultant to parents and friends with kids seeking wise advice—much to their peril, I should add. You will see what I mean.

Though I tried to avoid the title and function—I was the "expert"—psychologist-to-be, speech therapist, and special education teacher, I was *it*—the only person available!

When I was offered the "position" as special education teacher and speech therapist at the hospital (you've already read about that on a previous floor and chapter), it wasn't really a position—more an on-the-fly creation of an unwise hospital administrator or medical director (I wasn't sure which), and, of course, the Elks Club, which had adopted the hospital and scraped up the $300 a month for spending money for me. They offered me free room and board, living above the hospital in a nice room with a bathroom, and that walk-around money from the Elks. Sold! I accepted.

Wow. It was all I needed: a "job" and a place to live away from Dad's octopus reach, three meals a day, and something to do with my time making interesting trouble in psychology. I had no debt, owned a paid-for old car, wasn't married and had no children, and had a wonderful golden retriever dog named Duke (I've told you about him already).

Life was good. That was until the shock hit of what I was to observe and experience with these terribly sick, handicapped, and at times deformed by disease children. I thought I could handle it but went into a kind of shock at the emotional reaction I had. It was a psychological storm that took several months for me to weather. But I stuck it out, and it became an amazing blessing to me and my life. I'm glad I did. Sometimes I look back on those days, and I wonder if I could ever retrieve or somehow relive that happy simplicity. But no such luck or fortune.

There were many victories and crazy happenings my three years there, with a special treat during the weekends when I got to spend time hanging out with the orthopedic residents who were completing their child orthopedics surgery rotation from their various medical schools around the West (that is when I wasn't enjoying the company of the many nursing conferences and the pretty young nurses who sometimes stayed at the hospital).

I also spent various week and weekend nights as a waiter at a local steakhouse picking up extra spending cash and getting to know the locals. I also met a special tennis-playing lawyer buddy who told fascinating stories of his former life as a mercenary gun-runner pilot in Africa (it reminded me of a favorite movie of mine, *Secondhand Lions* with Robert Duvall and Michael Caine). We had crazy fun together as well.

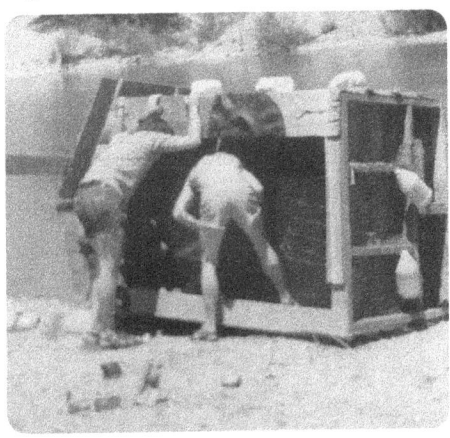

One time, he and I floated down the Rio Grande in an old desert outhouse (here we are pushing it into the river). But there was a nest of black widow spiders in it, which, startled by the cold water, began streaming out looking for the cause of their rude awakening. It was the annual town raft race with essential beer ice chest left intact, but outhouse boards broken off and floating their separate ways down the river to the finish before us. Did we finish the race? I'm not sure. My buddy's body may still be floating in it somewhere, and my apologies to his family for not searching more thoroughly.

Back up the hill to the children's hospital, I got to be very close friends with several of the surgical residents on bike rides, when horseback riding, and during parent consultation, as I mentioned. I remember learning the lingo these special docs at the hospital used, cutting my teeth for my future training as a specialist in behavioral medicine, my field-to-be. "What does FLK and FLF mean on your progress notes with my kids?" I asked. I was told FLK means "funny-looking kid" and FLF "funny-looking foot." They had their own special language so as not to offend anyone with writing these things out in the record. We do the same thing in psychology, but mainly in a lazy attempt not to have to write the whole diagnosis out, word for word—for example OCD, NSSI, ADHD, or ASPD (look them up).

The Hospital Kids
The hospital kids could also be unknowingly funny. I used to like to greet and talk with kids who had come to the hospital for treatment or at one of the frequent evaluation clinics, and one little black boy really tickled me. After finding out his name and where in the state he was from, I asked him why he was there at the hospital. His very confident reply: "I have SICK AS HELL ANEMIA."

Now most of you readers have gotten the extra humor here. For those of you who haven't—a common disease especially in African Americans is called sickle cell anemia—a pretty serious condition that is not curable and comes with much pain during episodes and flareups. It's not fun. I tried to keep from laughing out loud at his sweet but funny kid self-diagnosis. He was quite proud, and he should have been, that he knew the diagnosis and declared it to me in a loud, happy voice.

But the humorous times, which were many, did not assuage my initial trouble in adjusting to this new environment, its sights, sounds, and smells. I was completely unprepared (if one could ever be) for the profound shock and emotional struggle that hit me within the first week at the children's hospital (my two previous vocation- and life-affronting shocks came when in sixth grade I fainted upon dissecting a bloody pig's brain—no medicine career for boy John—and later nearly fainting during a clinical psychology training rotation in the hospital burn ward, with the smells and sights of severely burned flesh and excruciating pain in the patients. I don't need to explain that, do I? Thanks.)

The little girl's horrible condition was called progeria, and made her look 100 years old, with missing rotted teeth, leather-hardened skin, and tragically hard-to-look-at facial deformities. It's a rare syndrome that causes children to age extremely rapidly, and my first look, and those after for about a month, caused me to look away and even try avoiding her in the hall. I was ashamed that I didn't seem to be able to look at her except at a glance, much less to approach her and say hello or have a conversation—which I eventually was able to do. It was like a shock I was unprepared for, but I refused to give up. She deserved love and respect and I was determined to show it to her.

She was only about 10. I saw a number of other children with very upsetting diseases, almost as hard to look at. I was at first relieved the progeria girl was not sent to my classroom, but after some time, maybe a month or so, I was able to look her in the face and talk with her. It was a victory of sorts for me, and the loving, respecting treatment she deserved. I never forgot her.

I think I, as a newbie "child psychologist," experienced a similar kind of overwhelming stress a parent of a sick kid feels all too often. But I overcame, mainly by not quitting and gradually desensitizing to the traumatic things I would see. Then there were the wonderful kids too.

Michael

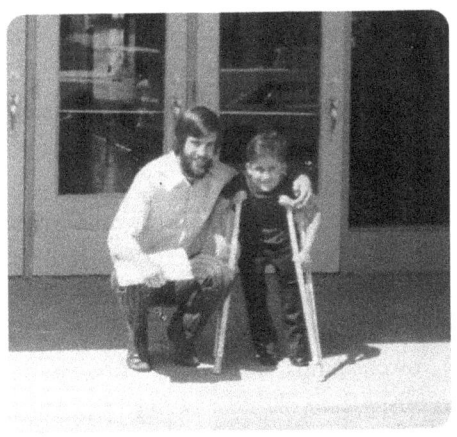

Another kid I fell in love with was named Michael. He had a condition in which he was born with his spinal cord separated and gaping out at the small of his back, rendering him unable to use his flaccid legs. He had an enlarged head and spinal fluid in his brain. You M.D. readers (are there any still reading?) will know the disorder.

Michael was a funny kid, whom I came to enjoy being with and teaching. During our months working together, a special thing happened to him. His legs were amputated. His parents and the surgeons decided to remove his highly dysfunctional, flaccid legs (which caused medical problems due to frequent infected pressure sores on them) and replace them with a series of prosthetic legs—starting with little baby ones. I have this wonderful picture of Michael on his tiny rocker starter legs, miniature crutches tucked under his small arms, standing between my legs. It's one of my favorite pictures that always touches my heart when I find it. I'm still looking.

Michael was in my classroom learning to read. He was eight and should have learned by then, but there was some mental disability that held him back, and he was never sent to school due to his life-endangering conditions. I'll never forget trying to teach him numbers. I would have fun with the numbers in order to help kids remember them, and when I taught the number eight, I told him, "This is Mr. Eight. He *ate* too much." He learned that pretty quickly, but there was a downside to my creative teaching brilliance: whenever I would show him the "8" flash card and ask what it was, he would always say "ATE TOO MUCH!" with great enthusiasm, hands shooting airward to accentuate his excitement at getting it right. It was funny at first, and we would laugh together. But I never could get him to drop the "too much" part. My teaching was too brilliant. After a good while trying to get him to drop the "too much," I pretty much gave up, hoping someday he would unlearn my silly memory scheme, and that today he doesn't still call eights, "ate too much." If you are Michael, his parents, or someone who knows him, and reading this, my sincere apologies if this never changed. *Mea culpa.*

My teaching creativity and brilliance took other turns, like when I discovered this amazing, color-coded phonics program for reading instruction. Great, a new tool! Let's use it! So, I implemented it in our little end-of-the-hallway hospital classroom. All went well, with certain colors equaling certain vowel sounds, *until they had to read in black-and-white—but they couldn't without the color-coding!* The more salient cue was the color and not the shape of the letter and vowel.

I think I set many kids back with this stupid reading program, some of whom may still not be able to read without colors. Another sincere, groveling apology is due, and I hereby submit it to all my former students and non-readers, waiting for those promised books written in phonic colors. Maybe I could create that business and make lots of money with those kids who still can't read except when colors for vowels are used.

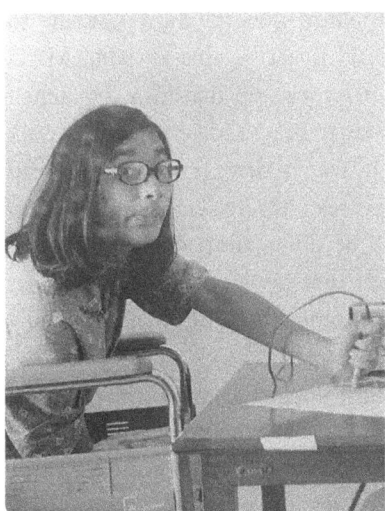 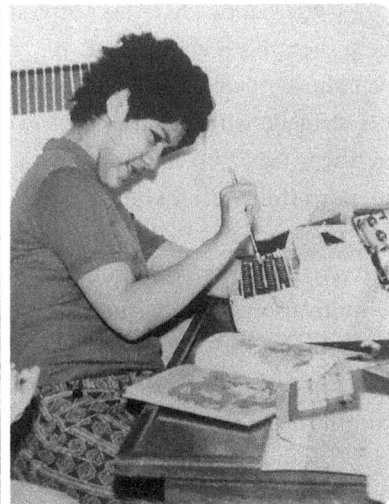

Maria and Isabel

These two wonderful young women were my first two students, even before Michael. They were a little older, teenagers, and they both had more severe forms of cerebral palsy (CP), including spastic and athetoid types. Neither could walk and were often told by their physician specialists at the hospital that since they had not been able to as children, that they never would. Maria seemed to accept that fate and remained in her wheelchair, but Isabel refused. She was bound and determined to walk if it took all her life! It was a kind of inner psychology and drive I had never been close to, or understood, and Isabel made a believer out of me.

Maria's form of CP was frankly more disabling, and her poor legs and coordination would not allow her the potential that Isabel's stronger legs and coordination had. I developed a sweet and caring relationship with both of them as their special teacher, and one time I was able to go visit Maria in her simple mountain home with her parents when I was nearby on a backpacking trip. She was special to me and I to her (I think she might have had a crush of sorts on me—and why not? A handsome young single man that I was!). Isabel didn't. One out of two wasn't so bad.

I was happy that the hospital medical director didn't ask me to help them both accept that they would never be able to walk. Maria was already there, and Isabel would *never* give up that idea. I watched her struggle with her full-leg, heavy-duty braces, determined to walk in them however dysfunctionally. It was a drive I had never seen so powerfully. Here's an informative test: try to *keep* a child from learning to walk. I dare you. It can't be done, short of some kind of a severe disabling condition, and then that person will *still* try. It was a motivational hardwiring I never forgot watching and ultimately encouraging.

I mostly worked on speech and language with the girls—a communication disorder was typical in CP where the motor (and speech) areas of the brain were damaged usually from a birth injury. It's hard to tell your tongue where to move when it just won't cooperate. Try making words, much less sentences, in that case. (Remember sweet Blanca, my first psychology "project"? She had a severe form of CP as well.)

I also did some teaching, reading and math and things, as both had not ever been in a normal school. This was a time when schools were not mandated to take these special needs kids, and in their districts they were not allowed to go. The hospital was their school and had been for quite some time. Things are different now, and our program and hospital played an important role in "forcing" schools to eventually take these multiply disabled, special needs students, sometimes under threat of suit. I was so gratified to have been a part of that important deinstitutionalization movement for the multiply handicapped and disabled.

Behavior Mod Guy

Nevertheless, and partly because of my work with these special students, even still completing my master's degrees, my "fame" was growing as a young hospital "psychologist" who could make kids learn and sometimes behave. Free psychology help from one who was not yet a psychologist! After a while, the reputation went on steroids when I performed that "miracle" with that screamer kid from the postsurgical rehabilitation ward (remember that kid?).

Bad Child-Psychologist Buddy

Following the sundry successes at the hospital, my fame and stories continued to spread. However, you will see from the following why we psychologists are strongly cautioned (and sometimes barred) from working with close friends and especially with family. The hospital staff had been watching me especially after the screaming kid with the "knee-monia" (I couldn't help myself there). They took notice, as did my friends, the orthopedic residents.

Charlie, a resident in orthopedics and a bicycle rider from California with whom I used to ride into the mountains on my bike, sat down one afternoon with me and kind of sheepishly (can a doctor of orthopedic surgery actually be sheepish?) said, "Can I ask you a question? How would you train an 18-month-old child to sleep in her own bed and not always our bed?" So the discussion commenced. Child psych 101. I was the teacher, he, my M.D. orthopedic surgery friend, the student.

By the end of the conversation, I had laid out a very nice behavior modification intervention. Or so I thought. This was easy peasy stuff. I sternly warned Charlie that he first get his wife on board for this plan, or it would be doomed to failure (and he as well, maybe). They had tried it the normal way by putting her in her own bed in the adjoining room, saying good night, only to find that the lovely little daughter made it 30 seconds to a minute before she broke down the parents' bedroom door with a baseball bat and demanded they move over and make space for her in their bed. Okay, she didn't do that. She didn't need to. (You will learn more about this in my section coming up on brat and nag psychology, though I think a child needs to reach the three-year-old threshold before the "brat'" diagnosis can be formally made.) It didn't help that this was a new second marriage and Charlie was the fresh stepdad. Uh-oh. Mom (number 1) and child (number 2) are in charge for sure. Charlie was number 3. (He knew, hence the sheepishness before me.)

This otherwise sweet little girl had set up her own, unauthorized squatter's camp in the parents' marriage bed, and would not be evicted, sheriff's order or not. Wisdom, expertise, and strength of resolve were required—by both me and the parents. The plan was to decide, commit to, and then explain to their daughter (together, of course, to avoid that divide and conquer strategy that all kids learn) that it was time for her to sleep in her bed all night—but that Mommy and Daddy were right there, and they would leave the lights on for her. Finally, this is the hard one, to not let her back into bed with them *no matter what*—except maybe in the morning when all were awake. Period. I prepared him and Mom by proxy for possibly up to a couple weeks of crying at night, but nevertheless to stand fast—even if it meant holding his wife down (gently) to keep her from going in to rescue the daughter (with the wife's written consent, of course—for legal purposes, you know).

So, he did that, she agreed, and all was well. Except that the next morning after its implementation, Charlie came rushing up to me at breakfast and told me, "Boy, are we in trouble." (We?) "I did everything you told me, my wife was fully on board, and sure enough our little girl carried on for most of the night, crying and weeping and begging. I had to hold on tight to my wife to keep her from going into the rescue and intervention breakdown." Charlie understood the significance of this trial for future child behavior control (and wife respect). He said some of her screams (the daughter's, *not* the wife's—though maybe both) were pretty scary.

To put it mildly, it was a failed experiment when Charlie approached me the next day with this dead-serious look on his face: "John, *your* behavior modification is dead forever in our house!" I think his wife won the battle of the bed, as did their darling daughter

Veterans, Trauma, and PTSD

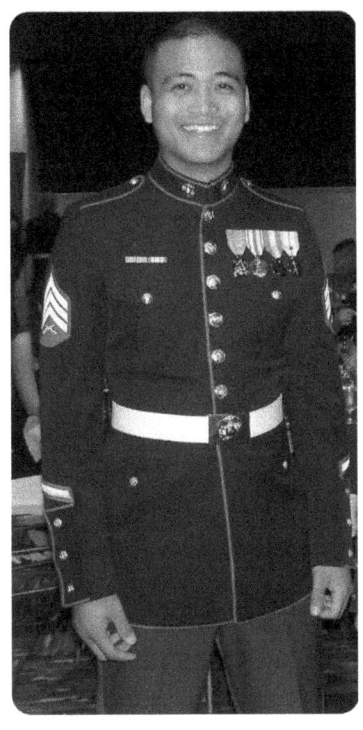

Gerry's trauma consisted of a combination of growing up in a harsh environment and family chaos, and experiences while serving his country. He would get triggered, traumatically, when he felt he or a friend (like me!) was threatened in some way. His response was to react in kind, even violently.

Profound psychological and behavioral "triggering" can occur suddenly and unpredictably, and that was certainly the case with him. One time we were riding bicycles down a city street on a lane dedicated for bikers, and a very nasty pickup truck driver and his evil girlfriend cut me off and yelled at me for getting in their way. My Marine buddy sprang into threat-mode action, caught up with them, and banged on their window in a very aggressive way. They pulled over, as did we, and threats were exchanged on both sides. I even got involved in the shouting and had to hold my friend back. I was eventually successful in getting the driver and his girlfriend to leave, perhaps by telling them my buddy was a Marine and a trained killer (I'm not sure I said "killer" but that would have been good), and that I could not hold him back from beating the two of them badly. It took us both a number of minutes to calm down after having been triggered in our respective PTSD.

One other even more severe episode occurred in an argument with his firebrand wife, half his size. At that point, he was not yet diagnosed with PTSD. She was trying to help him cope with his emotional sadness and anger that he was frequently experiencing. But he easily became provoked by confrontation or stress. During one disagreement with his wife, he was violently triggered and grabbed a knife. Police were called to the scene to de-escalate and he was later taken to jail. Unfortunately, this was not the first time they were called. While sitting in jail, however, he was seen by a mental health expert who treated him there. Eventually the VA hospital was able to take his case and get him the help he needed. As with many situations, his did not get solved by being in jail for one night. There were still months of separation and years of counseling. With the help of friends, family and church, the legal court system, the VA and bible group meetings, he was able to be held accountable for his actions and also get the help he needed.

Today, his PTSD is under much better control with the triggering episodes of fear and anger much less frequent and severe. He has other health issues, but he continues to stay in community. He and his wife both worked hard to get where they are now, and I tell them frequently how proud I am of them.

Due in part to his high-stress provocations and PTSD's traumatic triggering, his "poor choice" of parents (kidney disease went in his family), and his related higher blood pressure, he developed severe kidney disease. Today he is on dialysis and the waiting list for a kidney transplant, which he should get soon. We are all praying for him; in the meantime, commendably, he is leading two men's fellowship and Bible studies from his church. Such a great success! (His new kidney will come soon too.)

For many of our warriors, heroes, and first responders, it was their strength, toughness, and courage, accounting for their reluctance to talk or share, that helped them to cope and live even with the psychological and emotional "virus" that did not easily release them. But this kept it all trapped inside, which allowed it to infect more and more parts of their lives, their health, and their relationships. This kind of classical (Pavlovian) conditioning characterizes and explains PTSD, and fortunately there are a number of conditioning and exposure-based therapies that show promise and have brought many to restored lives. More recent clinical and brain research suggests the importance of brain "resetting" through brain, body-based, and mindfulness therapies such as EMDR and ITMS/TMS (intermittent/transcranial magnetic stimulation).

My most recent work with veterans with PTSD has included two exceptional men who lived in other states, and my evaluation and treatment of them was conducted remotely over the internet through secure video conference websites. It's known as "teletherapy" and is a new tool for treating a variety of psychological and behavioral disorders that previously required personal, face-to-face contact for working together and is now including PTSD. The results of my remote therapy for both veterans has been quite promising, bordering on highly successful.

In one case, his PTSD was so severe that he was confined to his apartment most of the time and could not even take a shower because of his panic reactions to being enclosed in that small shower stall space. Other features of his PTSD included helplessness and abuse from mistreatment by commanding officers, as well as profound grief over the loss of a chief under him.

When we began discussing his trauma, even before implementing the exposure-based intervention, he broke out in a terrified sweat all over and had to stop the relaxation breathing because (I concluded) it was associated with one or more of his traumatic events and reactions. I told him his powerful physiological reaction was actually encouraging, because his fear reactions were easily triggered, which would facilitate our work on therapeutic exposure, trauma processing, and desensitization of the fear reactions. I'm not sure he believed me at the time, but he trusted me enough for what I was saying.

We are now addressing and systematically training in rapid relaxation, body-mind calming methods, and then "walking through" the various trauma events, reactions, and fear stimuli as we progressively counter-condition and move toward extinguishing or significantly reducing and managing his terror reactions and triggers. An additional aspect of his PTSD has been the unresolved grief over the loss of his chief, under his command, whom he became extremely close to, and then who committed suicide. Depression is so much part of the military experience of trauma, and our armed forces members have one of the highest rates of suicide.

Nevertheless, despite the more complex trauma that has overgeneralized to his whole life, we were following the clinical adage:

"hurry the process, not the client." Effective treatment of PTSD should not take years, as some believe and have taken, but more like weeks and possibly months, if conducted competently. It can be done.

The other vet had experienced multiple losses and abuses during his time in the military, including the death of his fellow soldier and fiancée when he was not allowed to be with her. He had undergone harassment by fellow soldiers and his commanding officers, in which he could not escape or respond. It was that classic learned helplessness I discussed previously, and in combination with the blocked and unresolved grieving of the loss of his fiancée, and his former self and hope for his life, his depression and anger associated with his PTSD would overwhelm him. Because of his courage, never-give-up attitude, exceptional learning, processing, and desensitizing of many of his traumatic triggers while facilitating his grieving, we were able to reach the point of engaging the next step in our healing work together—the brain work.

He is currently undergoing TMS (transcranial magnetic stimulation), one of the newest and most promising brain "resetting" treatments for depression and PTSD, at a major medical school facility. Thus far, the results have been so outstanding for my client and many others that the VA is now including TMS as a therapeutic option for veterans suffering from these conditions. For my client, nearly after each session, he reports experiencing a profound releasing of stress, anger, and even grief as he continues to practice the mindfulness processing and exposure that we had worked on for some months previously through teletherapy. It's a powerful combination. The picture looks so bright for him that I have discussed TMS with my other teletherapy PTSD naval officer, once he is recovered enough to consider traveling for this additional treatment either through the VA or a major medical school psychiatry department.

Trauma experiences that qualify for a diagnosis of PTSD can be from life trauma, for example, growing up in dangerous, threatening environments and conditions, like my defending bike-riding Marine buddy. One individual I remember from a group at church I was helping to lead—an anger management group—told the story of having to call 911, the police, to keep him from trying to kill someone at a gas station who had triggered his traumatic rage by merely looking at him the wrong way. I talked with him after the group sharing and asked if he was in therapy or treatment, and if he had been diagnosed with PTSD. He had not been diagnosed, amazingly, and the therapist he had been seeing for about six years had never diagnosed, addressed, or treated him for trauma and PTSD. Withholding my outrage at that incompetent therapist, I told him what I thought he had and encouraged him to consider getting treatment for PTSD and possibly change therapists to someone who knew what he or she was doing.

Our veterans and first responders, as well as others with PTSD, can be encouraged that this is not a disorder that has to be lifelong. As I've noted, there are a number of evidence-based treatments that have demonstrated positive effects in reconditioning and desensitizing that profound alarm reaction to remembered traumas and perceived (but not actual) threats, including EMDR, CBT, mindfulness meditation, body work and PT, and TMS/ITMS. There are even brain stem analgesic injections that have shown promise. I will let you look those up if interested. There's lots written on them.

Part of my helping these veterans, many with old, undiagnosed, and untreated PTSD from WWII, Korea, and even Vietnam, included giving talks at veterans' groups and retirement homes. Of course, I would bring my service dog, Barnabas, along with me. Sometimes I think he was the one they wanted, but I had to be invited to come along and bring him. He would lie there up at the front beside me as I shared our experience helping the many vets with PTSD we had worked with and for. I've been asked to preside over memorial services as well for veterans who have passed on, and bringing Barnabas along is an understood condition (many of us have seen the moving scene of President Bush's funeral service with his wonderful dog lying there by the coffin on display in the US Capitol).

Sometimes in my talks before these veteran groups with my dog next to me, I would tell about some of my own struggles with PTSD, not from war zones of the military, but from family and other "war zones." I will be telling you about that in the upcoming chapter and floor tour.

But I'd like to make a final point here about PTSD and mental illness before we move on. Not surprisingly, some (including the veterans who have it) have described PTSD as a ticking time bomb, just waiting or on a hair trigger to going off or blowing up, possibly in a violent rage. It can be a constant, energy- and life-sapping struggle to keep these emotions and triggers under control and contained. Stuffed. Like a volcano, waiting to erupt. While relatively rare, violent outbursts may go over the line of violating others' personal safety and the law in general. Recall the anger management group participant who had to call 911 to get the police to come protect a person who had looked at him wrong, and my first PTSD client back in 1977 while I was an intern at the VA hospital, who beat up a whole bar full of people, including a police officer. Closer still to me was my bicycle-riding "wingman," who had pulled the knife on his wife and gone to jail, and then nearly got us both in a huge street fight, arrested, and thrown in jail. (I don't want to think about what my licensing board would have thought of that, not to mention the embarrassment of my friend's wife having to bail us out of jail!)

PTSD, like other mental illnesses, is not usually associated with criminal violence, but our military vets have been trained to react to perceived or actual threat in a warrior-like fashion—more from the "fight" and not so much the "flight" or "freeze" function of the 3 Fs of the sympathetic nervous system's threat response menu. This has caused many problems in these affected vets and to those around them, including domestic violence, road rage, and fights, among other criminal offenses. Now, this important concern brings to mind how psychology is or should be involved in our criminal justice system when mental illness or disorder becomes a criminal action or reaction.

Before moving on to my sharing some of my *own* personal trauma experiences and struggles, I decided to attempt to address this highly controversial area: How do we, or should we, deal with mental illness, including PTSD and our veterans, and the issues of guilt, responsibility, and punishment for those who have a mental illness and commit crimes. This is something in which psychology and psychologists, as well as psychiatrists, are often involved—*not* as mentally ill lawbreakers (please)—but as professionals and expert evaluators, witnesses, and treatment providers. As a society, as well as in our profession of psychology, how can we blend or somehow combine justice and punishment with compassion?

The following Can We Talk? is my attempt at this difficult subject. I will understand if you do not agree with me. There is much room for passionate and compassionate, but reasonable, debate.

> **CAN WE TALK?**
> *The Psychology of Lying, Guilt, Criminal Responsibility, Punishment, and Mental Illness.* Let's start with lying, confession, and guilt. They kind of go together. By the way, did you know that the lie detector, or polygraph, test is no better than chance at exposing lies and liars? It's true. Lots of research demonstrates this. So, flip a coin. But the courts won't. It's why lie detector tests are not admissible as evidence in a court of law. But it makes for good "entertainment," if you can call it that, on criminal investigation shows and *Dr. Phil* (though you especially should know better, Phil, being that jury selection expert with the court TV series based on you (!)—and stick to the good your show otherwise does, in educating, providing, and encouraging people with solutions to their psychological, relationship, and behavioral problems), and then there are those so-called reality TV circuses, like *The Jerry Springer Show*, with their polygraph exam truth-telling "fun," not to neglect the special added beating-you-up-to-get-the-truth test.
>
> Our friend Albert had the best answer to my question when I was teaching about "conscience" one Sunday service. I asked how can you "beat" a lie detector test: "Tell the truth? Albert concluded with a question. Way to go Albert! Simple intelligence rules! But that is too simple for too many.
>
> I once had a conversation with a police detective about lie detection tests that they frequently use. I thought I had him when I told him about the research on their inaccuracy, that they can fairly easily be beaten or fooled,

especially by experienced liars, criminals, and sociopaths devoid of conscience and emotional reactivity to lying. Then, he got me back: "*You* know that, and *I* know that, but the *criminal* often doesn't know that; we get more confessions on tape during the lie detector test or shortly after than you can imagine! (It's legal for the police to lie about the lie detector results—a wonderful irony, no?—to extract an actual confession from the suspect or "perp.") He won. There are better ways to tell whether a person is lying, but that's not my point here. I have a couple others related to lying and true guilt, having to do with justice and punishment.

Punishment vs. Rehabilitation. I once heard a very smart, highly educated, and obviously caring radio interviewer argue that the main purpose of the justice and prison systems was to rehabilitate the criminals and inmates, and that we needed to spend much more money on those services. I sent him an email stating (kindly) that he was an idiot (no, I didn't say that). I said he was wrong. The main goal of the justice system is, after determining guilt, to administer punishment appropriate to the crime—(hopefully) swiftly and surely—and *not* to rehabilitate the convicted criminal. And the punishment should be strong and effective enough to make the prisoner not ever want to do it again as well as hopefully convince people not to commit that sort of crime. Remember the definition of punishment—to reduce or eliminate the behavior it is applied to or associated with. Right? A further part of justice and punishment is to protect society from the reoffending-prone criminal by locking him or her up. (though some brain-dead city government officials have tried *paying* chronic criminals for *not* committing crimes! Idiotic. When, by the way, do we law-abiding folks get paid for doing likewise? I got it: never)

Thus, rehabilitation is not and should not be a primary (or even secondary) function of the justice system—that's not its job—but only a possible add-on that a compassionate society might choose to provide in helping the person not reoffend and become a law-abiding citizen, including things such as job training, personal and relationship counseling, psychological and behavioral treatment, and even non-government program help like the wonderful Salvation Army rehab programs, Bible studies, and Prison Fellowship that buys and takes Christmas presents to inmates' families and their children.

Does this all kind of make sense? I think so. But there's more, and I'm now getting to my main points regarding mental illness, criminal guilt, and punishment.

The Mentally Ill Criminal. But what of the person who commits a crime, especially a heinous one (like murder, for example), but is mentally ill? Isn't it the simple job of the justice system to determine guilt or innocence (actually, non-guilt, since none of us is innocent, if you get my drift) and decide on and invoke an appropriate penalty or punishment? Yet, guilt of a crime is a matter of fact. Did you do it or not. Period. But it's not that simple, is it? We have something called *"mens rea"* ("the intention or knowledge of wrongdoing that constitutes part of a crime") written into our law, which means if a person did not know what he was doing, or that it was "wrong" (or illegal) at the time of the crime, then he could be declared mentally ill, or having a mental defect, face no consequences, and go free. These folks who were presumably mentally ill (and might actually be so) can plead "not guilty by reason of insanity, mental illness, or mental defect" and be found *not guilty* for that reason alone—independent of whether they actually committed the crime—and then go free, bearing no guilt or responsibility for their actions. On one level it kind of makes sense, to be caring and compassionate. But on the other, it makes less sense. And how about the victims of the crime who experience no justice at all? There is no penalty or responsibility for the harm done to them or theirs. It doesn't seem fair.

I have a problem with this, even though it is the law. But how about the following alternative: pleading (or being found) *"guilty, but mentally ill"*? The person was or is guilty of committing the crime, as a matter of fact, but there are reasons that should be considered when compassionately and effectively administering punishment and the overall sentence. In the case of those pleading or being found guilty but mentally ill or with mental defect, their sentence can include time, treatment, and therapy while incarcerated, until such a time as their mental illness has been successfully treated, and possibly resolved—after which time they serve out the remainder of their sentence, or are re-tried, or their sentence is modified on compassion grounds. I know, how could I be so non-empathic and cruel?

But compassion and justice need to work together, one after the other, with compassion following (not leading) guilt, accountability, responsibility, and punishment, in their proper order. Perhaps some, or too many, have gotten off "scot-free" after committing even terrible crimes, because of brilliant lawyers who know how to work the system using and manipulating the *mens rea* defense—to their client's joyful escape from all punishment, accountability, and responsibility. It's a tough one on both sides, isn't it?

Evil. But where does or can evil come in here, whether you believe there is such a thing or not? Like when a person, a serial killer, commits such horrendous crimes against others, with no conscience or remorse? Scott Peck, M.D., has written a book (*People of the Lie*) about this, suggesting we create a diagnostic classification in the next *DSM* (6 or 7?) for "evil"—the next category, significantly beyond that of sociopath, psychopath, and ASPD, including the most severe pathological signs, symptoms and prognoses, and, presumably, the most severe punishment matching the evil of the crime. Now I'm not arguing for the death penalty here, but one could. Anyway, I found Dr. Peck's arguments persuasive. Maybe you might too.

Just sayin'.

ROOM 502

PERSONAL TRAUMA CONFESSIONS

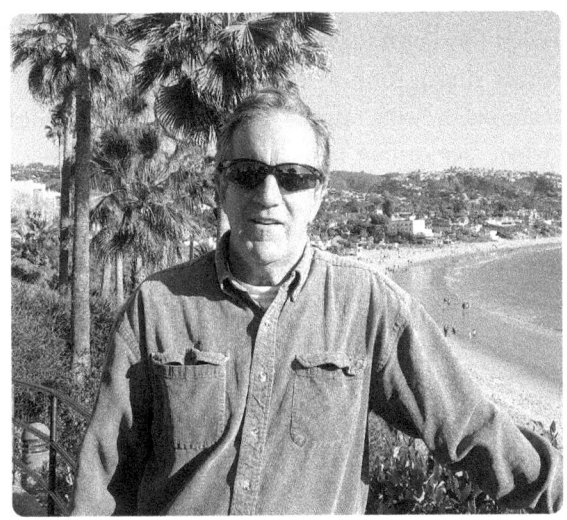

"Knowledge is power."
—Francis Bacon

"A little knowledge is a dangerous thing. So is a lot."
—A. Einstein - F. Bacon - A. Pope - (pick)

My path to psychology was directed in some real ways, and ultimately engaged out of my childhood and early adulthood traumas. Trauma had a significant effect on me as a redefining and dictating life factor. Trauma explained much about me, and ultimately my direction and approach to my life and career. My educated guess: virtually all of us have faced trauma at some time or another in our lives. It's what effect it has on our lives and how we have dealt with it that makes the difference one way or the other.

Trauma can be defined as an event that is potentially overwhelming, psychologically, emotionally, and maybe physically—that invokes the survival reflex—the classic "fight, flight, or freeze" response. It's hardwired into our brain and psyche. We can't help but react, often with great and lingering fearfulness and psychological triggering and breakdowns—like the veterans back from war zones with the deepest form of trauma, PTSD.

I remember during one of my many trips to Africa, this time while on an animal-viewing safari, I asked the African guides what one should do when face-to-face with a lion, not to mention a charging lion. They gave me two responses. One I understood, kind of, and the other was completely lunatic. First, you cannot outrun a lion. They will catch you and eat you. I learned later, a male lion has a 35-foot leaping ability, from a seated position! At one lion farm where a raised walkway permitted close observation over the electrified fence, we were told if you fell over the rail, the lions below would catch and eat you before you hit the ground! I didn't need convincing.

But then came the second answer: your only chance is to run straight at them. Say what? Are you crazy? Run toward a lion? Actually, no creature charges at the King of the Beasts, certainly not a weak (and tasty) human! A crazy person, surprise attack is the only chance you have. But I was warned, you will probably still be eaten. Oh, thanks a lot. But freezing in fear was the only other option, though not such a good one either.

I once read in an airline magazine on another trip to Africa, a story about a group of men from Mozambique. They were sneaking into South Africa at night to find work on a trail the lions knew well and would lie in wait for them. Seeing the lions, the men froze and didn't move or speak for a number of hours. I think it was six. The lions got bored and walked off, sparing them. Amazing. But if you can't stand motionless and absolutely silent for six hours, then running at them is probably your only hope. Lions can represent the threat and traumatic fear we sometimes encounter in life—either suddenly, as on a battlefield, or chronically, growing up in a toxic family or dangerous places like parts of Chicago or LA.

Even though we don't generally face lions, all other kinds of threats can be equally or even more traumatic. Our brain is wired to respond rapidly to any perceived or actual threat, especially for survival. When the alarms go off in the emotional and cognitive centers, we must choose to run, stay and fight, or just freeze in fear or feigned death, like the deer in the claws of the mountain lion in hopes it will loosen the grip temporarily so she can flee. It happens. But when we are unable to run, fight, or adaptively freeze in order to run later, the trauma goes within. Our brain internalizes the stress in our emotional, psychological, and memory areas, where it all can get embedded, possibly infected, and maybe become toxic.

While adults may be able to reason with a trauma threat and take rational action or inhibit the reaction and calm the alarm when it is not a real threat, children cannot. Children are especially vulnerable to profound traumatic reactions that can include terror, or pathological depersonalization or dissociation of themselves with the trauma and reality. It's a defense mechanism that can have long-lasting, damaging effects behaviorally, emotionally, and psychologically.

I've seen a number of clients who had had these profound traumatic experiences and reactions affecting all parts of their lives, and I did too. I was one of those children and young adults critically affected by trauma, which had a life-crushing effect on who I was, my relationships especially, and my life directions. I experienced three significant traumas during childhood, and one during my late teen years, such that my life was anxiously driven and powerfully redirected and redefined by them. Let me tell you about them. Perhaps you might relate personally to one or all of them (I hope not, for your sake), but even if not, they may be worth the telling here.

Trauma One: Abandoned and "Killed"

The first one occurred when I was four years old when my (formerly) loving parents told a huge lie to my one-year-older sister and me, as they dumped us at the hospital in New York. They told us we were going shopping. They didn't want to buy us toys and things, as we imagined, but rather to rip out those four uninvited tonsils without our consent or permission! We were tricked, and the doctors, nurses, hospital, and our parents were in collusion in the grand deception! Okay, a little hyperbole there, but looking back it seemed true, through nobody needed to go to jail. Call it a misdemeanor (but a bad one).

We were abducted, not taken to a store, but to a big monolithic hospital building, and *abandoned* without a word of explanation. This was the "old-school" philosophy and practice pushed ignorantly and seemingly uncaringly (toward the kids, not parents) by the medical folks, probably to avoid any stress to the parents and doctors, no doubt, not the children captives. "Just don't tell them what is going to happen, and leave. We will take it from there. It will be less stressful if they don't know what we are going to do to them." It's different these days. Children are taken for a tour around the hospital environment, maybe even including the operating room, and one parent likely stays overnight or close by at the hospital.

These complete strangers, dressed in weird clothes, bad people really, took our clothes and shoes, gave us these funny gowns, locked us behind bars (bed cribs), and then, sans (formerly) loving parents, left us completely alone, abandoned. Adding insult and trauma, I was separated from my sister, whom I didn't see until after her ordeal. I was wheeled, separately, into this big room with a huge bright light and strange, scary people again peering over me, everyone in masks. The next thing, a killer man pressed this big black rubber mask over my mouth and nose and tried, successfully, to suffocate me! I fought, but they won. I died.

Resurrected somehow from that black hole of death, I came to. But that night, I awakened spitting blood (stitches broke), and the whole terror happened *all over again*—double trauma and abuse. Three days later, my parents "gloriously" reappeared, all smiles, with ice cream and a new drum set for me. It wasn't enough.

I had nightmares for many years about that terror in the big white "store" with the suffocating, "killer people." I think maybe this trauma had much to do with my fear of going to sleep. It didn't help when Dad explained to me when I was a bit older, and curious, that when you die it's just like going to sleep and never waking up. It was related to my bedwetting until after I was 10—a very late age for a child to still be wetting his bed. The doctors, and especially my parents, never apologized. The night terrors that continued for years and the stress-related bed-wetting signaled the beginning and incubation of my PTSD.

There is a well-cited psychological study conducted with year-old babies, called the "blank face" study, that powerfully illustrated the profound, psychologically traumatic effects on babies of parents physically and emotionally withdrawing—going blank—from them, even temporarily. Like abandonment at the hospital, my tonsillectomy trauma was this study on steroids.

Speaking of my trauma-imposing mother and father, they were pretty serious drinkers, probably what we would call alcoholic, and I wondered later if many of our emotional needs for safety and comfort had been neglected or ignored, sufficient for the blank-face abandonment effect. Nevertheless, Dad was so convinced that our family was "perfect" that he refused family counseling even after a high school counselor was so worried that she made a strong recommendation that we all come in for help. So, of course, we didn't go. "They were the crazy ones, not us," he stated.

Somewhat ironically, Dad's heavy drinking (It was "perfectly" social according to him, reminding me of the definition I once heard of a "social drinker"—one, who when around other drinkers, says "so shall I.") resulted much later in two serious bouts of pancreatitis—an acute life-threatening medical condition. The first attack caused him to miss my marriage; he couldn't come he was so sick. The second came perilously close to killing him.

I was at home with him visiting when he experienced his second and more serious pancreatitis attack. He woke me up late one night in a real crisis. He was pale and sweaty, dry heaving, and feeling very sick. I took him to the hospital, and it wasn't long before he was diagnosed with pancreatitis—his pancreas was inflamed (due to chronic drinking almost without question), and his digestive system had shut down. It is a serious, potentially fatal condition, and it was fortunate that the IV antibiotics pulled him out in a couple days. They kept him in the hospital, but the crisis was over, and, released, I traveled to see a colleague and friend of mine—incidentally one of the world's experts in alcoholism treatment. When I explained to him what happened to my father, I shared that maybe I should look for a good time to possibly confront him about his drinking and the dangers to him.

My colleague's response was classic motivational interviewing: "Let me see if I've got this right. Your father is in the hospital after a nearly fatal bout of pancreatitis that is due to his chronic drinking, and you are wondering when would be a good time to address this with him?" DUH, JOHN. I got on the phone, called family, and requested a meeting with his doctor in the hospital room to confront Dad. The doctor was a "keep the peace" sort and he was a very reluctant participant—not wanting to upset the old applecart of his relationship with Dad, who "needs to have at least one or two vices to enjoy life." But I insisted and threatened. We assembled around Dad's bed a couple days later. I conducted the family "intervention," and I prompted the physician (I might have kicked him under the rolling hospital patient table) to tell Dad that even ONE MORE DRINK COULD KILL HIM. What was so hard about that to say? Apparently, it was. But the doctor spit it out, and Dad heard our pleas for him to stop drinking because we loved him and didn't want to lose him.

Here is where Dad's stubbornness actually worked for him and us. He refused to let me pour out all the bottles of liquor at home before he was discharged, and soundly rejected the idea of AA. His answer to my questioning was this: "When I make up my mind to do something, I do it." STUBBORN. Argh. But he did and lived another 15 years more thanks to that stubbornness, our "intervention," and the doctor's threat. Victory.

Night Terror
One of my night terrors, seemingly connected to my death experience at the hospital, consisted of my body becoming stone cold below my neck, like what actual dying must feel like. My fear of losing control, and of blood, both seemed connected to this fear of death. Looking back, I wondered if this nightly terror as I released into dying darkness

and twilight sleep had as much or more to do with my other profound trauma—one of the classic signs of sexual abuse as a child. My body parts would go numb, especially in sexual areas below the neck. It was a psychological protective or defensive mechanism we call dissociation, when a person disconnects in the deepest way psychically, from a most profound trauma that a child especially cannot understand or cope.

Trauma Two: Sexual Molest
This one probably had the most devastating and long-lasting effect on me and all my relationships, especially my attempts at marriage. But then again, what did I know. I just knew what happened later in life by my symptoms and did a sort of retrospective diagnosis.

I was sexually abused and molested as a young boy, and possibly as a baby. The evidence for sexual abuse grew to a breaking point following having an emotional meltdown the day after I married my Christian sweetheart. When I should have been filled with joy and love, I was sucked into a pit of darkness, depression, anger, and withdrawal for two weeks. This pattern repeated almost every time within three days of making love, according to my wife.

This got both of our attention, and I sought therapy with a trauma expert in another city but wasn't able to continue. Nevertheless, I began to look at my history of symptoms and childhood memories—including a nearly complete gap in my childhood memory before about 8 or 10 years old—and contacted my mother in an attempt to confirm what seemed to be sexual abuse or molest as a young child. I had all the classic symptoms. In many ways this was the most insidious and profound, because it was hidden from all of us, and especially from me, and in the 1950s this was neither a topic of discussion or of much interest.

As I mentioned, the first notable symptom was that I remembered very little of my childhood before about 9 or 10. It was a dark space, and not normal. That alone is diagnostic, and my shyness and social insecurity probably masked a resulting childhood depression, anxiety, and withdrawal, continuing into adulthood.

When I had to look at my symptoms and began to investigate, my mother told me that she remembered her concern over two situations.

First, my kindergarten teacher, a man, was caught having his students including me sit on his lap in ways that even got the attention and concern of parents and the school (at a time when there was little or no focus or understanding about child sexual abuse). Second, my mother noted that there were signs of strange, concerning behavior toward me by our maid, housekeeper, and childcare person, including one day when they found me with her. My clothes looked like they had been carelessly and rapidly put back on (inside out) when they came home suddenly. While my memory was blank for that period of my childhood, my signs and symptoms powerfully pointed to sexual molest.

It all added up: my symptoms of intimacy terror in marriage, my body dissociation and night terrors, the highly suspect kindergarten teacher and maid behavior, and nearly a complete block (repression?) of childhood memories—all pointed strongly to sexual abuse in earlier childhood.

Interestingly, the field of psychology learned that Freud was probably more right than not in his initial diagnosis and reporting of child sexual abuse in his Victorian women patients who struggled with psychosomatic paralysis. In addition, our understanding of multiple personality disorder (not schizophrenia, which is not multiple personality), now termed DID or dissociative identity disorder, can be due to early childhood sexual abuse and molestation. I seemed to fit there as well.

Child Trauma Three: Father Abuse
Trauma doesn't have to be from a single incident or several similar events, like we see in many of our military veterans I've seen for PTSD evaluation and treatment. It can be what we term complex trauma, which can occur from a chronically stressful environment or conditions imposed by others, such as living with an abusive parent.

My father never beat me, but he might just as well have. It would have been more obvious that way, and at least more understandable. The verbal and emotional abuse was more hidden and insidious, the type that can be hidden from others, and from self. Dad was one of those classic Type As, driven, highly competitive, impatient, angry, hypercritical, even mean. What hid it, and complicated this picture, was his charm and humor, which I've already related to you. He was a complex abuser, self-made man, highly successful, and prideful. I vowed never to be like him and became almost exactly like him. That is, until my spiritual transformation.

I remember my wife sharing a story about me as a dad to my wonderful five-year-old son. When he wouldn't obey her, she'd asked him, "Why do you obey your father, but you don't obey me, your mother?" His response: "Because I'm *afraid* of my father." I laughed when she told me that, not considering the unhealthy fear of my temper and occasional yelling around the house.

I never ever dared to back talk my father or to utter a swear word in his presence. I was afraid of him—later finding out I harbored a hatred, even rage at him. I finally summoned up enough courage for the first time ever as a 30ish psychologist on the faculty of a medical school to talk back to him, objecting to the way he constantly criticized and put me down. He was so shocked at this display of standing up for myself and in opposition to almighty him that he called my chair at the department of psychiatry to find out what was so terribly wrong with me! Humiliating.

Dad's Type A heritage and abuse affected me deeply but was kept underground for a long time until I was in therapy after my marriage failed and I ended up in a "family sculpture" role-play exercise. In it, I was on the "hot seat" and had to designate people to "play" my family members and tell them about them. I placed the dad model up on a chair, towering over me. I then was led by the evil therapist (she made me talk with everyone), one by one, down the family tree. When I got to the dad guy, I was powerfully overtaken by a rage that frightened the guy, the group, and me. I would have tried literally to beat him to death if he had so much as touched me or said the wrong thing in our conversation. This so freaked out the group, and the therapist, that they shut down the group. I don't remember going back, but I do remember walking around for days, upset at what happened and seeing that cancerous rage in me surface and frighten us all. I had no idea.

I even developed a type of phobia, called misophonia, or hatred, even rage, against others' eating sounds. Maybe you've experienced that mild irritation when especially obnoxious people are eating near you with their mouths open, like loud popcorn eaters in a theatre or someone slurping soup—but that's not it. It's more extreme. Rather than causing a slight irritation, a kind of emotional rage or hatred takes over, traumatically, and it's all you can do to keep from yelling at the offender, or wanting to hit them, or run screaming from the place. Sound crazy? But I figured it probably had more to do with a conditioned aversive reaction to the association with my father's loud and obnoxious eating—as we all sat silently at the dinner table listening to him, in fear and anger after his latest blowup and verbal abuse of our mother or us. I only learned there was a name for this so-called disorder a few years ago. I didn't know anyone else had that problem. My wife will tell you what it's like trying to eat around me.

Trauma Four: LSD Horror
The developing brain is highly sensitive to trauma, even through adolescence and young adulthood, and can according to a growing body of scientific study, literally rewire the brain in certain ways. When the trauma and brain wiring and misfiring has the added insult of a drug-induced hallucination, it is like trauma on steroids. Have you ever seen the Ad Council's public service commercial warning us of what drugs do to the brain, showing the egg frying in the pan on the hot stove? Then you get the idea of how certain substances can "fry" the brain. That happened to me and my brain.

I was in college, a stupid 19-year-old freshman (would that be redundant?), and took LSD. I had a horrifying "bad trip" that lasted three days and changed my brain and life, presumably forever. I appeared to have experienced a traumatic, psychotic break with reality during that hallucination-induced state. It was my fourth major trauma on the road to insanity and ultimately PTSD.

I went insane that day. It was a day, and a single fateful decision, that sucked me down the wormhole of insanity. Psychosis, or more specifically, a psychotic break, seized my mind and ultimately life after that. I became suddenly and profoundly unbalanced, and it took many years and psychologizing energies, experiences, learnings, and (mis)directions in my attempt to rebalance myself. Before: insecure, relatively happy (or so I thought), kind, good sense of humor, and adventurous. After: traumatized, hallucinating, anxiety disordered, flashbacks, withdrawing, angry, hyperreactive, hateful, and mean. It led me away from what was seemingly normal to the abnormal, and to my quest to find out what had happened and what was so terribly wrong with me—to psychology.

It was the spring of 1966 when I first thought I had gone insane. Not at first, the trauma of my scrambled mind all too overwhelming to deal with, but later, as I crawled back to barely enough sanity to decide I had indeed. It was an episode that polarized me and drove me into a psychological world of horrors. I was a stupid freshman (once again, redundant) in college, away from home. Without much sense or forethought, I took LSD. I had heard about it, I think. It was actually morning glory seeds laced with strychnine, I'm told, that had a similar effect to LSD. Maybe worse.

I was handed several of these "pills" by a fellow freshman in my dorm and was told they would make me "high." Cool. Not really. I was the only one who took them who didn't vomit. It all went to my brain, unfortunately. I spent the next two days in my room, hallucinating, terrorized. If I could have killed myself by throwing myself out of the window, I would have. I couldn't move from my bed. I saw blood and dragons and serpents. I had no idea where those images came from, but they were terrifying. I thought I was going insane. In many ways, I had.

After those three terrifying days in my room, I managed to function, barely. I'm not sure how I kept going to classes, and I do remember going to see the campus psychologist, who helped some but not much. All the psychiatrist could offer was a tranquilizer, which I didn't take. Nobody understood or believed, and I stopped asking and talking about it even to the few with whom I tried. I figured I had a profound break from reality. I didn't call it that then but do now. I just knew I had gone crazy. It only confirmed my fears when I almost immediately started having flashbacks of the horror I experienced those three days in my bedroom.

I will always remember the first terrifying one. I was sitting in the dorm cafeteria, eating roast beef, potatoes, and gravy (an important detail). Then it struck. The flashback. All the memories of the hallucinations came roaring back, and I had my first panic attack. I thought I was dying, a defining symptom I later found out in graduate school in psychology. Nearly paralyzed, I found the residual energy to rush out of the cafeteria and run up to my room. I think I stayed there for days before coming out. I developed agoraphobia, or fear of crowds and enclosed spaces, with panic, and would have attacks at least once a week. I didn't have a name for it until years later, when I diagnosed myself—agoraphobia with panic, and later PTSD. I just knew it was terrifying.

Phobias and More

My self-diagnosed agoraphobia with panic did not stand alone. I had other phobias, or near phobias, that caused some paralyzing effects and resulted in my missing aspects of life, fun, and especially loving relationships. If the circumstances and my fearful reactions were not sufficiently controllable, I learned to avoid. I guess becoming an expert in clinical psychology was a part of that avoidance. The more I knew about it and could intellectualize, the more controllable it seemed, and I became quite good at avoiding those things, circumstances, and people that triggered those fears. Sometimes I would sabotage the relationships in my life that triggered my fears. Linda was one precious relationship I fearfully destroyed, and I missed out on so much more. I know there are others who have experienced similar reactions and coping efforts. You too? Hopefully not.

> **CAN WE TALK?**
>
> Multiple Phobias, PTSD, or General Anxiety? Can one have more than one phobia—that irrational, nearly all-consuming, overwhelming fear of something or some situation—or even a series of them? Sure, why not? Maybe the more you and I have, the less there is to go

around for other people in a zero-sum world (sorry: another of my stupid humor attempts). But they are a serious thing, especially for those who truly suffer and may be disabled by them.

Let's say there are three phobias or extreme fears stacked together somehow. Would that be a *psychological trifecta* or *tri-phobia*? I'm not aware of this unique diagnosis in our manual, the *DSM-V*, but perhaps there could be. Case in point: I had three that I eventually self-diagnosed and managed to turn from disabling phobias to extreme fears, or panic, when all efforts to avoid them failed:

(1) *agoraphobia, with panic* (my fear of bustling, noisy crowds, open places, and being too far from the safety of home—starting with my LSD trip and flashbacks imprisoning me in my college dorm room for days and weeks),

(2) *acrophobia* (my fear of heights from teenage years, including desperate plague-like avoidance of those moving "death traps" like Ferris wheels, roller coasters, huge swaying buildings like Taipei 101, not to mention canyon precipices and hotel outdoor glass coffin elevators!), and, as if that wasn't enough,

(3) *claustrophobia* (including the ultimate death trap terror—the enclosed MRI tube. I once panicked inside one, demanding to be let out, with nightmares about being stuck in a dark small cave or well, arms trapped, facedown). I once laughed seeing a cartoon of a woman, in obvious panic, about to be put into an enclosed MRI tube, as the Dr was explaining how they needed to get an MRI to find out the cause of her claustrophobia. Stupid.

Do you relate to any of these? I hope not, but suspect you do for at least one. You pick.

Now, being a bright guy, I became pretty good at avoiding those situations—despite my son's accusation that I was a "chicken" when refusing to go on those harrowing #2s or choosing (huff, huff) to take the stairs rather than ride the hotel glass coffin elevator death traps. Avoiding walking along the edge of cliffs, or the tall building or hotel overlooks was pretty much candy. The rumbling Romanian salt mine actual death coffin elevator was not easy to excuse myself from, especially when coaxed by pretty ladies in our party.

But maybe these fearful reactions could have been a type of generalized anxiety effect or disorder, I surmised, from my more primary traumas and then PTSD. A feature of all phobias and PTSD generally is that overwhelming fear and panic from death or impending doom triggered powerfully by some familiar or reexperienced stimulus, memory, circumstance, or event. If so, you, like me, could qualify for something called GAD, or this generalized anxiety disorder.

But the theory and treatments are quite similar for each and all—GAD, anxiety disorders, phobias, and PTSD. It's a generalized learning or conditioned reaction from any perceived threat or actual aversive stimulus. We can be like Pavlov's and Seligman's dogs (remember the cats escaped, but the dogs stood and took their "medicine," so to speak) and those things even loosely associated with the fearful thought, stimulus, or event—invoking the same intense overwhelmingly fearful response. You know, the survival mechanism reaction kicks in and the brainstorm of fight, flight, or freeze along with it. You are in the threat and alarm side of the (mid) brain when you really need to be in the calming, rational side of the prefrontal cortex. Unfortunately, when you are reacting out of the threat and alarm mid-brain emotion flood, the forebrain function needed to calm and reason with these false or irrational threats is "offline." Fortunately, there are ways to switch your brain focus from threat to calming reason, such as with something called EMDR (Eye Movement Desensitization and Reprocessing). It was very helpful for me, but not enough space to explain it. Look it up. There's lots written on EMDR and its companion, mindfulness meditation and awareness.

Recovery or a form of healing can also include (a) natural desensitization—letting time and general exposure to those things wear down or out the fear response

> when nothing bad actually happens (this can take quite some time on its own); (b) programmed systematic desensitization or exposure therapy, which strategically pairs those triggering stimuli with a more relaxed physical and emotional state; (c) medication to modulate the anxiety and fear reactivity (being careful, hopefully, of the potential for addiction to the so-called minor tranquilizers and anti-anxiety drugs); (d) other kinds of physical interventions such as directed brain stimulation (TMS), analgesic brain stem injections, or even, more recently, (e) therapeutic administration of hallucinogenic drugs such as psilocybin. I'm not sure what I think about this last one, but the therapeutic "barn door" has apparently been opened with new clinical findings reports suggesting its efficacy in some cases. Have you heard the phrase: "Time heals all wounds"? Unfortunately, mere time heals little in the way of psychological and emotional wounds—only physical wounds. But methods all the way from (a) to (e) can go a long way towards this kind of healing, or at least functional recovery.
>
> *Suggestion:* If you have an anxiety condition or disorder, phobias, or PTSD, like me, but as yet untreated or not successfully resolved, don't give up. We know much more about those conditions. In fact, we now have a number of evidence-based treatments and interventions. Sometimes things as apparently simple as body-focused relaxation or tension release can help immensely—such as massage, yoga, tai chi, etc., especially when performed in a community or group (you've probably seen the tai chi folks in parks, especially in Asia). These body movement-related forms have been found to be more effective than psychotherapy—for example, in a study on post-911 trauma and PTSD in New York. They've worked for me too. Definitely worth a try.

The PTSD Fight—More Trauma

My "recovery," or at least thick-headed persistence, was sufficient somehow to pull me through two master's degrees in psychology and speech pathology, and subsequently the Ph.D. in psychology. It wasn't until I was well into my professional walk as a psychologist and professor that I discovered that I had PTSD. Nevertheless, the LSD trip alone didn't seem to warrant, much less explain, my PTSD symptoms, so I began looking at my past before college and uncovered those four major traumatic experiences that fit and seemed to qualify. And one common aftereffect that can overwhelm or at least delay one's recovery is when we are triggered and retraumatized.

Retraumatized

I experienced two traumatic kinds of flashbacks, or re-traumatizations, that were related to my PTSD I believe, and reminded me of the seriousness of the emotional cancer I had carried for so long. Both had to do with emotional rage. As many traumas and PTSD perform, a type of flashback can be triggered, and I was not immune or recovered sufficiently to avoid those occurrences and recurrences—hard as I tried to suppress, avoid, or deny them.

Father Rage

The first happened when I was in that group therapy program following my divorce and I had that profound rage reaction against the group member who was "playing" my father in a type of family role play. I had no awareness of a rage toward my father previously but thought later it could have been related to my past traumas. It led me to individual counseling that helped, and a letter asking and giving forgiveness to my father.

Airport Rage

The worst was when I was going through the TSA airport check and was singled out for a pat down. It was early 2015, post my academic career (but not my full healing, apparently). I willingly submitted to this unkind treatment on a trip to get to my flight with my friend and business partner. The TSA agent was doing his job, but when he got close to and maybe even touched my privates, something profound took over. A *rage* welled up inside me, probably a protective dissociation related to my childhood sexual molest, and I went into a traumatic hypnogogic state.

I stared angrily at this man who now had become an evil enemy and told him loudly, three times, "GET YOUR F---ING HANDS OFF ME NOW!" In my rage, I was prepared to beat him to death if he didn't. This was not a rational choice, as if I had tried, or even laid a hand on this man, I would myself have been beaten, shot, and if not killed, thrown in jail. Probably by the grace of God, I did not attempt to kill him (I would have), and he stopped and passed me through.

My business friend and collaborator on our development of an on-line motivational treatment program for depression, Vip Patel, was in shock at what he had just observed. As I came to my senses, I attempted to explain to him what happened. For three days, I was unable to sleep because I was so profoundly (re)traumatized. When the colleague and psychologist friend we were visiting heard about my episode and reaction, he encouraged me strongly to get treatment, even suggesting some evidence-based therapies that could help, including the newest, TMS. I actually sought and received benefit from one of those, EMDR, and hope to try the TMS therapy as well, though not as significantly needed.

Interestingly, research on brain and body functioning related to traumatic reactivity has pointed to the importance of the body and physical components feeding into the stress reaction. We therapists help to teach the kind of body and mind relaxation, before exposure therapy with the traumatic memories and stimuli, in a form of counter-conditioning desensitization of the triggering stimuli. A most fascinating study of trauma victims of the 9/11 attacks in NYC seemed to confirm this—finding that the most helpful therapy for these first responders and others was *not* psychotherapy, but those things that had to do with body relaxation and calming, such as massage and yoga, where there is physical touch, and ritualistic movement such as tai chi, especially when done communally.

Traumas Six to Ten: Cancer

Many of us have suffered from the trauma of cancer, whether directly or indirectly.

Insidiously, cancer is a trauma that likes to hide, often just until it is too late—leaving its death grip on not only the cancer victim, but also upon those loved ones around him or her. I remember seeing a poster in an AA meeting hall that relates: "You don't have to drink to suffer from alcoholism." Similar for cancer. Significant personal loss can and often does cause trauma, persevering traumatic reaction, even full-blown PTSD. What's more, the caregivers and medical professionals can have lasting trauma reactions that drive them out of the field. Case in point: one of the highest burnout and turnover rates is found in nurses working in cancer wards. The losses there are daily and profound.

Besides experiencing childhood and young adult trauma personally, cancer devastated our family, like it does many other families as well. For me, the count was five plus one: grandmother, mother, sister, fiancée, best friend, and wife. I lost three family members, one fiancée, and a best friend to cancer, and nearly a wife as well. These losses were understandably traumatic, not just to me but to the family. They are losses you never really get over, and they had an enduring and further traumatic effect on my path to healing and hopeful recovery.

Though I found alcohol and marijuana as useful "helpers" in my numbing out my traumatic reactions, they both turned on me. I found shortly after discovering marijuana and hash that I would experience a retraumatization of fear of loss of control and dissociation of my mind to my body—which would go fearfully "dead." So, I stopped. But alcohol was a different animal. I could control it better—or so I thought—and then there was the horror of nearly dying at 16 on a trip with an equally stupid buddy when I drank beer and bourbon all day, and then chugged nearly a bottle of VO Whiskey. I was unconscious for two days, lost all bladder and bowel control (that happens right when one dies, I'm informed). Why he did not take me to the ER is beside the point. That was another trauma that led only to my avoiding whiskey, not beer.

Marriage Breakdown

My marriages suffered the most from my various traumas and my PTSD, and combined to further the traumatic soul wounds of my life. Nevertheless, despite my marriage failures, I kept trying, maybe in an effort to heal myself, but always to no avail. I had a pastor friend once tell me, commenting on my persistent attempts to remarry, that I was either the most optimistic person he had ever met, or I was one of the most mentally ill. I think he was right on both counts.

From Trauma to Recovery

Trying marriage once again was not sufficient, with basically the same breakdown results. My significant romantic loves and ultimately relationship destructions spanned more than 40 years, from Linda in college through Lucia, 40 years later; but the marriage breakdowns had the most profound effects. All the same, I remained hopeful and kept trying, whistling in the dark as it were. The next marriage was supposed to once and for all heal me.

I believed finally that marriage to a beautiful, godly woman who had waited was the best I could have hoped. And it was. For a day. Then came the awful trauma drowning, this time worse than ever. I became afraid, then angry, then depressed, and I withdrew, she says, for weeks. Physical intimacy was a trigger, and I would "disappear" into angry depression and the stonewall of protection. It usually took place within three days of sex and could extend for a week or more. My wife kept notes on her calendar. It wasn't like clockwork, but more akin to a time warp, being dragged back into the child past never known, resolved, or reprocessed, as the EMDR therapist would describe. It was crazy. Efforts at therapy were unsuccessful, and we and I finally gave up. But a more profound thing had happened before that, leading me to believe that my issues would be smooth sailing ever after. The Spirit was healed, but not the flesh, as the Bible warns.

ROOM 503

TRAUMA COPING, THERAPY, AND RECOVERY

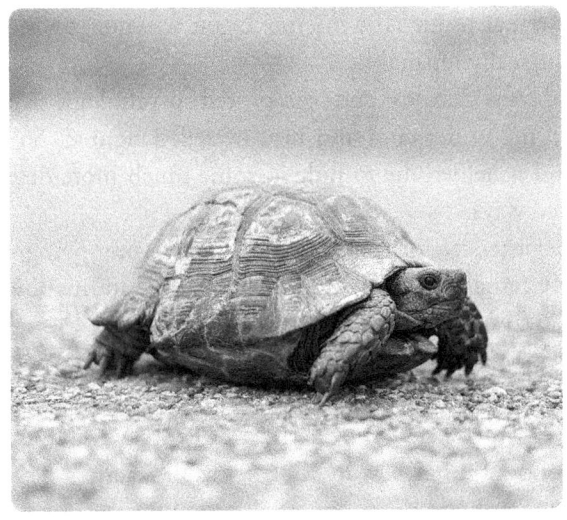

"When you find yourself in a hole, stop digging."
—Mark Twain

It was a slow road to healing, or at least coping, to achieve some semi-normalcy for me. It was like that of a tortoise crossing a highway, somehow avoiding being run over. I had to juggle my career, marriage, fatherhood, and my trauma dealings—not to mention road to recovery. In addition to marriage, I pursued many directions and made numerous efforts to deal with and heal from my trauma. But it was a cancer that affected virtually all parts of my life, and to cope I tried to hide, and then find relief in any way I could. But you don't heal cancer with aspirin.

Sports helped in my younger days, especially ice hockey (we lived in the north then), where I could vent my anger and rage as a part of the competition. My senior year in high school, I was starting defenseman and the most penalized player in the league for fighting. When I had surgery on my nose years later due to breathing problems, I was told by the surgeon that the bones of my nose and face were all crushed over one side of my face. Hockey fights. Go figure. My face bore the external brunt. The internal brunt was not so visible, not to mention surgically repairable.

Then I was led to and discovered psychology. Maybe that would help me understand and heal myself, I figured. So I made it a career, and it helped me to hide in some much more defended and sophisticated ways.

My persistence, or perseveration, kept me going—but not healing. My father once gave me a halfhearted affirmation when he told me I always finished a job I had started (I think he was referring to mowing or raking our two acres of wooded, hilly lawn—but no matter. I received the rare blessing). During my most difficult post-psychosis year in college following the LSD trip, I found music. I was not very good at guitar playing, but it was distracting enough, while driving my roommate nutty. But the traumas were cumulative, from childhood, traumatic floodgates breaking at my LSD-like, psychotic "trip," overflowing into every part of my life.

Reaction, Coping, and Road to Recovery

Indeed, the multiple traumas, especially those from my more vulnerable childhood, had a profound initial effect, followed by those further deepening and infecting ones. I was just short of a complete emotional and psychological breakdown and then breakthrough, as I weathered each further installment layer of trauma. It was like an onion, and when one layer of infected, traumatized experience seemed to be peeling off, as dead skin, another would surface and demand attention, whether I was willing or not. I was mostly unwilling.

I was accused of being a workaholic, burying myself in teaching, research planning and running, grant writing, and time with students and colleagues. On top of that, my additional survival mechanism was exercise addiction, running up to two-hour lunch breaks in every weather, 5:30 AM 15-milers before breakfast, training runs, and seven marathons including New Orleans Mardi Gras (twice), Mississippi (twice), St. George Marathon, New York, and Boston. I justified both as positive addictions (well, they were, weren't they?)—which helped me to avoid facing and processing the emotional wounds: fear, bondage, reactivity, depression, anxiety, and especially intimacy avoidance. They worked to delay and distract, despite the corrosive effect on my life and relationships.

I tried marriage to normalize and heal as I've said, but that did not work, and they failed mainly due to me. I tried achievement, and that seemed to work for a while, but not really. I tried drinking, and that definitely worked to numb me out enough to push on as a phony happy party guy. Then I had a go at spirituality, learning and practicing transcendental meditation (TM) for seven years, that is, until the day I "achieved nirvana," according to a Buddhist colleague, but it terrified me when I went so far inside myself and found only darkness, emptiness (and despair). So, fearfully, I stopped that. But I pressed on until the breakdowns emotionally, and then relationally, became too much.

Looking back, I'm not really sure how I managed to fearfully push on in life—not to mention pursue study and a career in psychology—given those traumas spreading viral-like from childhood, undiagnosed and virulent like cancer. Nevertheless, I survived, but just barely, it often seemed. Then I found the therapy I required: drinking.

Drinking "Cure"

I discovered alcohol starting from age about 14 or 15—that efficient, convenient balm for my emotional and psychic wounds. We know in psychology that it is the immediate and not the longer-term effects that predict and determine the behavior. Those more immediate effects almost "miraculously" helped me numb out, even temporarily forget, as many of my later veteran clients with PTSD would describe. It was that mostly controllable, artificial peace and happiness doing its intended job, calming my brain, emotions, memories, and hyperreactive triggering.

I loved beer. Drinking beer was not really drinking, I figured, not like those alcoholics down on skid row, or slouching, beaten up, in those downtown AA meeting halls. For me it was refreshment, a good socializing companion, friend, and fun enhancer. Drinking beer, you may know, is essential on the water while boating or sailing, which I did as often as possible. Seven sailboats and 40 years later, I still enjoy an occasional beer, but not like before. The need was different then.

Having a six-pack or two on a sail, or one after work and at parties, was no big deal, and certainly not a concern of mine. Besides, I never got that drunk or that often really, so it wasn't a problem, I rationalized. I was once confronted in a group therapy session as to the purpose of my drinking, not so much the quantity calculation. The numbers were fine. What could be the problem? So what if I had to have a few beers every day after work to "take the edge off," not to mention throughout the day on the weekends and at parties. Hey, it was only a few beers and not hard liquor.

I had tried pot and hash in college and after, for a few troubled years, but I didn't like the feeling of losing control that accompanied it—especially the more powerful blends that wrestled me across the DMZ separating the real, in control, and hallucination boundary. Losing control felt like dying, so I unnaturally avoided those things that were uncontrollably scary. Like the roller coasters and Ferris wheels I fearfully avoided after learning I never had to subject myself to this terror again. Drinking helped me to avoid and continue to suppress the emotional and psychological turmoil that wanted out, but that I wouldn't let out. Not until much later when, dam breaking, it gave me little choice.

My college counselor referred me to a psychiatrist when I came dragging there, terrorized and traumatized by my LSD-like hallucination trip. The psychiatrist didn't know what I was talking about, retreating to his Occam's Razor solution: medication. The universal "cure" for anxiety—nothing minor about minor tranquilizers. Benzodiazepines, the so-called (wrongly) non-addictive solution to anxiety disorders and even alcoholism. Later, the academic circles I lived in—teaching and health research—knew little about how to treat, much less diagnose, trauma and PTSD, that is, even years later in 1986 when I finally knew. It was ironic. I should have looked to my work eight years earlier with the military but did not. It was a blind spot, and a big part of me preferred being blind. My wife certainly didn't.

Alcohol was more efficient and there was lots of company. One wedding reception after a friend's wedding, I discovered champagne. It was sweet and bubbly, of course, and next thing I knew I was very happy, too happy. You know what I mean. This was back in the days when MADD hadn't gotten mad enough, and buzzed and drunk driving were the norm (in New Mexico then, you could drive through and purchase a large open beer as a driver). Stupidly, I was put in charge of bringing the wedding cake to the reception after the wedding. Driving my happy group of six friends in my car, arriving at the reception, they asked who brought the wedding cake (my group's simple task). I thought one of them had it. I certainly didn't. I put it on the roof of the car, so who put it in the car? No one. Retracing my route, I found that huge, sweet, creamy white slick covering the whole street. Oops.

Back to the water, I especially loved drinking while sailing—a requirement, I concluded, and followed that practice religiously. It was a great combination. That is until one Fourth of July out sailing with a bunch of friends on my 25-foot sloop (I forget her name)—and drinking lots. We (I) rammed the same houseboat twice that day. I was at the helm, of course, and who put that boat in front of me? The second ramming nobody in their boat came up on deck to see who had hit them. They knew. "It's them again! That same boat full of drunken people. Let's not antagonize them and just hide." There were other stories of beer and sailing that I won't bore you with. My son, Josh, and brother, David, can fill you in, though both had culpability as well.

Red Flag

My trauma at 16, almost dying those two days after drinking myself to death (and resurrection) should have been red flag enough. But it wasn't. I just gave up drinking that kind of whiskey—VO Whiskey—that tried to kill me and probably did. I've been quite successful avoiding it since then and have little taste for hard liquor—that is until I discovered on one trip to South Africa this amazing fruit liquor that elephants love and get drunk and wild on, Amarula. It's my wife's favorite and I brought a bottle back from our recent trip there. I kind of hoped she'd get a little crazy on it, like the elephants, but no such luck if you know what I mean.

So, I just adapted. I knew what I could drink and not drink and attempted to count beers just short of getting drunk, in order to avoid getting drunk. It's not the best strategy, shall we say. It's kind of ironic, trying to control the behavior that causes you to lose control and conscious awareness. I remember learning that alcoholism, or a more severe drinking problem, was not losing control and getting drunk even after a single drink *every* time—but it was the inability to *predict* whether or not and when you would get drunk. Thus, the person who can sometimes have a couple drinks and stop is not necessarily a person who doesn't have a drinking problem. If he or she is unable to predict whether drunkenness occurred, almost by surprise, some would say that points to a likely drinking problem, or alcoholism if one uses that term.

My parents were big drinkers. That seemed normal, as all their friends drank, and Dad would come home after work and have a martini or two or three, and perhaps after a two-martini lunch in the city. Weekends were work around our big yard—to which I was slave labor for—and then parties with their friends. I absentmindedly never paid attention to the times my mother was caught hiding gin bottles around the house (my brother did notice), and their liquor cabinet was always full and replenished when not. I found out a lot more when I was in treatment for my drinking some years later.

When coming to visit me at my first job, my parents arrived in the evening on a Sunday. When Dad discovered I had no alcohol in the house, and I lived in a dry county in the South (and it was a Sunday when "everyone" was at church, not at bars), he turned right around and drove over the state border to buy booze. I was shocked when he did that. It caught my attention, but I quickly forgot. It's curious when one buries or discounts personal or family evidence like that, which could help one's own understanding and possible personal healing.

After my second marriage broke down and failed around 1983, my drinking and emotional states got worse, much worse, and I became clinically depressed. The alcohol continued to do its job of numbing me and now it took more and more. But a loving friend of my ex, and recovering alcoholic like her, confided in me one day that he was concerned about me. He suggested that I reminded him of his own daughter who was a classic "adult child of an alcoholic," or ACA, and recommended I join an ACA group he was running. I agreed, and my more directed coping and recovery was begun.

The group was a bit of a shock to me. I was a clinical psychologist and professor and certainly didn't belong there, but I humored them and stayed. It helped when I discovered I fit every symptom and criteria on the ACA checklist, such as the terrible triple of "can't trust, can't talk, and can't feel" growing up in an alcoholic family. When the one-month group was finished, the leader, my ex's mentor, recommended I do it all over again. I guess I didn't get it. Angered, I nevertheless agreed. Where else was I to go? This included attending ACA and Al-Anon meetings, for those from alcoholic families, stopping drinking (even though of course I didn't have a drinking problem), and attending some AA meetings to see the real bad ones, of which I was not one.

After this second ACA group, it was recommended I attend a longer-term and more intense outpatient group. I knew I didn't need that but agreed once again. This group really let me have it, such that after about three months of my halfhearted attendance, they recommended I go into a halfway house for people in recovery. What? I was angry and almost walked out of the group then and there. But something came over me and I asked for their reasons. It hit me, like a sledgehammer to the chest: 1. "You need to be around others to transform your life"; 2. "You should stay away from any new romantic relationships"; 3. "You have a lot more to learn about yourself and changing your life"; and 4. (this was the hardest-hitting one) "YOU NEED TO BE HUMBLED!" I was arrogant and prideful, and angry and miserable underneath my thinly veiled phoniness of expert professor and fun-loving guy.

For about three days I wrestled with my anger, fear, and new knowledge, and finally decided to go to the halfway house. Vocational Rehab picked up the fee (what a great program that was), and I was dumped as roommate with a tattooed criminal from the state prison—probably for murder. He loved verbally abusing me and started from the beginning calling me "Doc"—spitting it out contemptuously when he spoke. I'll never forget his telling me to shut up in a powerful way: "Doc, if I was you, I would do a whole lot more listening and a lot less talking, and more getting with this program!" I was scared of him.

I had chores around the house, had to attend AA meetings regularly, move out of my home by the lake, and give up sailing for a while. I got to go to work at the VA every day, then back for dinner, meetings, and chores later, and on weekends. I wanted out but needed their recommendation first. Whenever I asked, I was denied, with the statement: "You are not ready. We'll tell you when you are." I was being humbled, as prescribed by the ACA group.

Roughly three months later, long after I had ceased to ask to get their recommendation for successful completion, came the conference with the home leaders: "You are ready to leave now. We now can recommend it." But I no longer wanted to leave. I had been humbled, developed friends, and was attending AA meetings with a new positive attitude. I asked how they knew I was ready. I know there were more reasons stated, but I remember one: "Because you no longer want to leave." A powerful spiritual transformation happened earlier in my time at the halfway house, which had much to do with my changes and readiness to leave and will be discussed later.

In the 12-Step program, I attended meetings almost every day, sometimes twice, or three times (!) on especially tough or lonely days (noon, 5, and 8 PM). In a way it was my first church, where I experienced unconditional love and acceptance. I know I am not alone in that feeling. I became a student of the 12-Step recovery program, *The Big Book*, and fellowship, as I attempted to follow the steps of change. I had two exceptional "sponsors" who helped me tremendously to transform and change. One led me through the steps yearly, and the other I watched in meetings for about six months until I got up the nerve enough to ask him. He was an African American who was filled with life and joy and would light up every meeting when he spoke. "I love sobriety!" he would gush, and the joy of his new sober life flowed over those lucky enough to be there. I timidly asked him that day if we could go out to coffee together to talk. He said yes, and no sooner had we sat down and he said: "Yes." I was confused. "Yes what?" I asked. "Yes, I will be your sponsor, now let's get started."

Stanley was an amazing guy, and I grew quickly to love him. One day when I was having trouble with a couple of the steps—especially the making amends step—he told me in no uncertain terms: "I want grandchildren, so if I am going to continue to be your sponsor, you *will* do these." And I did, with his help. Sadly, Stanley committed suicide some time after. He apparently had bipolar depression and it got to him. I'm sad writing this and believe I will see him one day again.

Despite the powerful help of the 12-Step program and fellowship, I needed more, and I tried whatever else I thought could help me, my anxieties, my depression bouts, PTSD, and my related relationship craziness. My reactions and efforts to cope with and recover from my trauma and PTSD included stopping drinking, following the 12-Step program, getting sponsors, "curing" my exercise addiction and my ongoing workaholism—the great professional distraction and ego "satisfaction" resolution! All worked for a while, singly and alone, and then not.

I tried forms of counseling (I *was* a psychologist, after all, so why not that as a last resort, dummy), but I was a tough client who knew too much—often more than the therapists or psychologists I gave the benefit of my company. I one time got up and walked out in the middle of a session with my wife, as the female therapist yelled at me (recollections of my father's yelling at his cowering son). No matter the device, substitute, or counseling attempt, there was never real healing or much hope, until I gave up trying. Strange.

I think the day I stopped all that striving was the day I began looking for true meaning and peace outside of and above me, and not the "nirvana" emptiness cure within or from external self and others' manipulations. Nevertheless, I continued to distract, numb, and avoid what truly needed to surface and be healed—my PTSD. Given my growing God-centered spirituality from the 12-Step program and meetings, I was pretty certain *God had other plans for me*. I just didn't. know what or how to get there. I pretty much knew I was worshipping at the wrong altar—psychology and "self"—"but did it mean I had to leave psychology altogether? And I guess this book is one of those results of hanging in there and making lemonade out of life lemons. Read on to see some of the details in that quest.

SIXTH FLOOR

PROFESSIONS—BEYOND PSYCHOLOGY

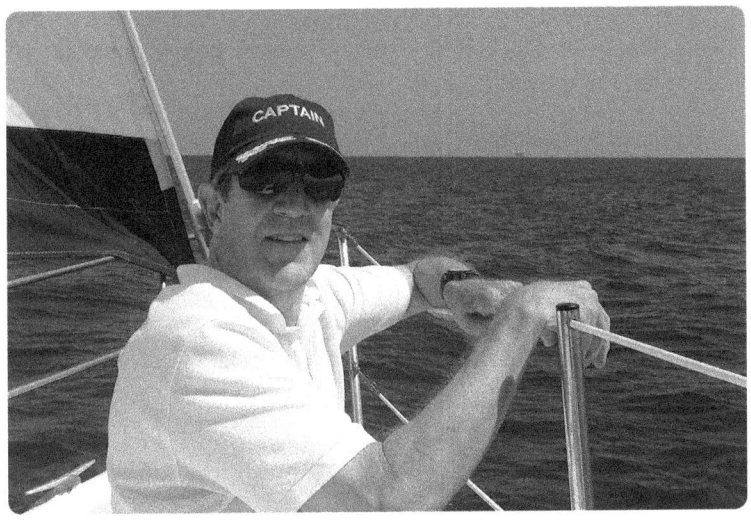

Captain John, out to sea - turbulent waters and stormy passage ahead.

*"[Find and] Be yourself.
Everyone else is already taken."*

—OSCAR WILDE

My profession in psychology evolved into the spiritual, and then the religious, in a life transformation. The sixth floor chapters trace what happened to me personally, professionally, and spiritually, and what I did with it. These were disparate, maybe even competing, roads that came out of my desperate state—roads that were not intended to ever be merged, and I had no training in how to deal with such a thing. I found out I couldn't separate or deny the three tracks—the personal, professional, and spiritual/religious—but nevertheless had to come to a decision about which way to go, the why and especially the how. My great conflict soon became whether and how to stay in psychology or go beyond or away from psychology—changing "professions."

You may have encountered one of these profound crossroads in your life, and especially in your career. In these chapters, we will see what happened to me, what I did with it, and why and how I finally decided to stay in psychology—to find a new, greater purpose, and integrate the three roads into one.

ROOM 601

THE PSYCHOLOGY OF HOPE AND FAITH

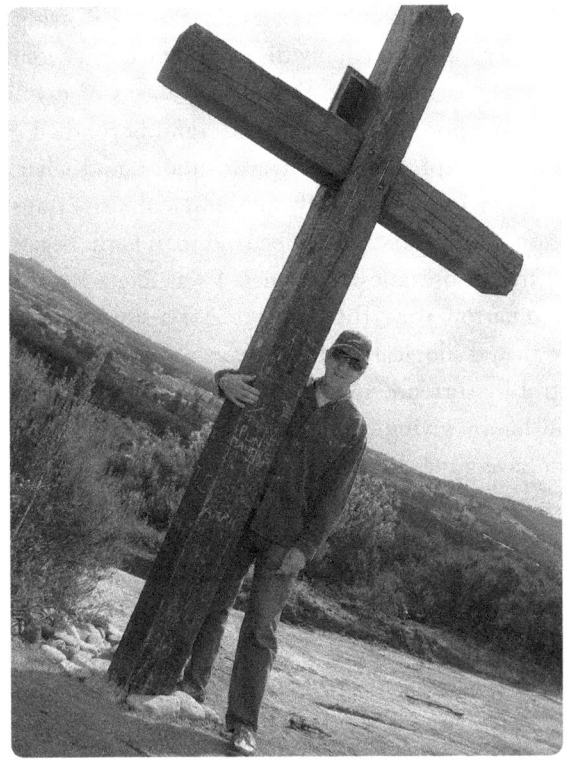

"If you seek me with all your heart, you will truly find me."

—JEREMIAH 29:13

The healing I desperately required had to come ultimately from that spiritual route, through faith, and a radical experience with

God. You know I was too hardheaded and arrogant to get it the way many do—they just decide and believe. I was the "puffed up with knowledge and without wisdom" kind. My transformation to come included certain coping relief like stopping drinking and hanging out in powerfully spiritual 12-Step meetings, but then evolved to reading the Bible after experiencing unexplainable miracles in my life, eventually leading to life purpose, peace, and service. It all roped me into my training and education as a pastor, leading worship and Bible study at a shelter for the mentally disabled (where my wonderful new wife and I were married). But I'm getting ahead of myself. Let me tell you about my finding hope and faith (and beyond). I guess some details would be helpful here for you to understand what happened and how and why I was powerfully (and miraculously) transformed.

To be honest, my pursuit of hope, and then faith, began internally out of my external breakdowns. I guess I was like a lot of other folks on that same narrow way. The path was not a simple, easy, or logical one. In fact, it was illogical. It didn't make sense to gain by giving up, to get control by surrendering, or to heal by breaking up and down. And to find life by giving it up. But that was what happened. Those of you who have gone through what a colleague has called quantum change, and all who have had a profound spiritual awakening know what I'm referring to. It's paradoxical, even when you can't find a pair of doctors who will diagnose it. (All right, I apologize, but we are now in the section on hope after leaving the dark one on trauma, so give me some grace here.)

Chaos Transformation
My final marriage breakup, my broken heart and ankle, drinking blowbacks, and clinical depression all led to the turning point, as the AA *Big Book* describes. When I discovered chaos theory, I finally had a kind of explanation. All combined to form a chaotic hurricane of swirling upending winds with no apparent eye or end. Chaos theory explains that any unhealthy "system" invokes a "self-healing" process that breaks up the rigidity to create a type of "healing variability." This happens when a system becomes so "diseased" that a type of rigor

mortis sets in and binds the system, person, organ, or relationship to a rigid and ongoing sickness and unhealth.

The system, person, or relationship, rigidly broken down, becomes vulnerable to some breakup of the sickness by an invading variable or intervention. It is like when we try to conduct a family intervention, confronting the sick person to cause a shakeup and change in a member's addiction. Profound change can then occur when this healing variability takes over the formerly rigid sickly system and produces that self-healing process, now liberated. We talk about transformation and profound, sudden change in a person—such as one with a drinking problem who suddenly decides to change and does relatively permanently, almost defying what learning theory or psychological science could predict, invoke, or explain. A study of this has defined it as "quantum change"[21] and attributes much of the healing process to a spiritual or religious phenomenon, according to those who have reported such profound and sudden change and transformation.

My breakdown, ensuing disease rigidity, shakeup, and breakup, and then quantum change had much to do with spiritual and religious factors and facts. For me, it was a road of finding hope when there was none, finding faith despite unbelief and resistance. It came not all at once, but in layers and waves, and then all at once. It is worth telling.

I was not a believer in God or miracles, and certainly not religion. My transformation and form of self-healing came not from church or church people—whom I avoided for obvious reasons—but from what the Bible calls, "the hounds of heaven" pursuing me. You might be skeptical, and so was I. See what you think after hearing what happened. I want to be careful not to make this book and story into a religious one—it is not—but to tell enough of that side of the story, surviving psychology and finding hope and faith, to enrich and explain only.

There had to be a spiritual "kick" that broke me out of my rigid depression and withdrawal from life, a powerful turning point that began from the bottom. The day I stopped TM initiated years of searching for other hope, not the internal kind. I was done with that inner pursuit.

But now I was depressed and afraid to get back to life. Then the unusual started happening. The first hope interruption was a phone call and what happened after it. Some would say "miracle," but the way I interpret it now is not important. My image at that point was like the old audio speaker ad showing the guy in front of the speaker with his hair all stood up on end in shocked frizz.

I was on my pity pot, as my AA friends would say, feeling depressed with little or no hope. My then wife had left and was with another man, whom she then married after divorcing me. The heartache was unimaginable, and it was the first time when I didn't care if I lived or died. There would be a second, final time too. Trying to jerk myself up from this dark hole, I decided I should stop this depressing, painful, and destructive self-obsession and turn my thoughts to others, or another, to get the hell (figuratively) out of the quicksand of the unholy trinity—me, myself, and I. I thought, maybe someone who was sick, with cancer or some life-threatening illness, who needed help. That would be someone I could help as a way to get out of myself. Then, a mere minute or two later, as I was marinating on this thought, the phone rang. It was the church calling, where my runaway wife and I were married. They were looking for someone to help, and for some strange reason my name came up, so they called.

I was too depressed to want to help and began to say I couldn't, when the church worker continued, as if not hearing my denial. There was an older man, a grandfather, who had terminal cancer, and he was at home to die and was too large for his frail wife to help him do things such as go to the bathroom or move around their home. I pictured of my favorite grandfather, Dukie, whose funeral my parents had not "bothered" me with as I was in college somewhere else. Realizing how my thoughts of what I needed to try to do had led somehow to this providential phone call, I changed my mind (maybe knocked to my knees at this point as I remember) and said I would help. I ended up staying with him several nights a week, all night, helping him to the bathroom or other places around the home. He was big and heavy, but I was young and strong. It and he touched my heart in a deep way. He died not too long after my time helping them. I suppose, actually hope, I will see him again one day.

If that was a miraculous call—the subject and timing of which was at least highly coincidental—then what happened the previous year certainly seemed to be. A little while before she left, my wife and I were having a pillow "fight" and one blow hit me square on the head like a hammer. The pain was intense, traveling down my neck and spine, and was unrelenting for about a minute. That was unusual and got my attention, especially since my neck stiffened up so much that I could barely sleep that night. It was with me the next morning and through the day at work. I found a neck collar—you know, the kind people wear to court or gatherings when they want everyone to know how hurt they had been—and wore it. Then, one of my more observant and caring residents under me at the hospital suggested quite strongly that I go see a doctor about it before I left. We were staff at a hospital after all. So, reluctantly, I did.

Ray was an orthopedic surgeon on staff at the medical school and friend enough for him to drop what he was doing that late Friday afternoon and attend to his psychologist buddy. Naturally, he wanted to get an X-ray, so I was promptly sent over to radiology for some pictures. The staff radiologists had left for the day, but there was a small group of bored, and then quite eager, radiology residents covering. When they saw the film, they got unusually excited. You know how a doctor looking at test results or an X-ray expresses excitement, it's not usually a good thing. And it wasn't.

Dr. Ray, viewing the film on his screen, thought I had a broken neck but didn't tell me at that point. He pointed out a black line crossing through one of my cervical vertebrae—the second or third one, I think. It was high and not good either way. "So," I commented, "I guess I'll just have to wear that neck brace for a while longer." Shocked at my comment, he said, "No, we may need to do surgery tonight. This is very dangerous, and you could sever your spinal cord if we are not careful. But I want to be sure. I need to get some more film and need you to go back." When I heard the words "fracture" (broken neck) and "surgery tonight," I stopped thinking—dragged into terror and fear. I think I retreated to the wall for support, to keep from fainting. I remember gripping it.

The second set of films popped up onto Ray's screen and showed the same: dark fracture line at C2 or 3. My terror continued, and he wanted to get one more series of X-rays to be absolutely certain, before scheduling surgery that night. I carefully walked back over to radiology, and lying terror stricken on the table as the X-ray was being completed, I said what I believe was my first prayer ever. It went very close to the following: "God, I will give you my life if you take this away from me and heal me."

The third set of films showed no dark fracture line. It was gone. That was impossible, I thought. It *must* have been a miracle. Dr. Ray probably didn't think so, as is common for doctors when presented with what appears to be a miracle healing. He said something about the X-rays somehow showing an anomaly that was due to a bad position or filming angle. I didn't agree. Profoundly relieved, I left his office, had a good night's sleep, still wearing the neck collar since the neck was still sore, and promptly forgot my prayer and deal with God—or whomever. But God didn't forget and put that prayer deal into the proverbial bank, for later withdrawal, I guess. I went back to my regular existence, plodding along, avoiding depression and retraumatizing events, until my wife, who broke my neck with that pillow, left me for another man. The hounds had been unleashed, and it was no contest: I tried but couldn't outrun them.

I remember a special television investigation show (I think *60 Minutes*) looking at the science of the Shroud of Turin—that piece of cloth that reputedly covered Jesus after his crucifixion. It caught my attention since the scientist interviewed was a physicist, and not a believer in God, who attempted to disprove its authenticity. But he and his team of scientists, despite a variety of sophisticated tests, could not. The blood and cloth appeared to be consistent with that age, and miraculously one might conclude the apparent image of Christ on the cloth was found to have a third dimension, showing depth—an impossibility according to the scientist's team. I remember walking around for some days struggling with that. Could Jesus have been who He said He was? I finally decided he wasn't, couldn't have been, and so I did a Steve Martin as the medieval barber Theodoric of York, contemplating whether they should use science rather than bloodletting leeches for healing a person. So I chose not to believe Jesus ever existed.

There were apparent miracles that touched my life, both before, when I was in college, and after my ensuing spiritual experiences and ultimate transformation. I had just broken up with my beautiful college girlfriend, Linda, and depressed, I did something I never did—I called home. My relationship with my father was not a good one, and I knew it would be late and probably wake him up. But walking through the library that night I had this powerful urge to walk over to the public phone and call home. I woke Dad up—I'm not sure if his wit engaged with a comment to my apology for waking him: "No, you didn't wake me. I was getting up to answer the phone anyway." We spent some time talking and he was unusually kind and understanding. I felt better.

I flew back home for summer vacation a couple weeks later and Dad picked me up at the airport. He told me that my mother was in the hospital after suffering a heart attack. She was in the ICU on a heart monitor with a pacemaker in her chest. When I called Dad that night after the breakup, he went down to wake up Mom, who often fell asleep in front of the downstairs TV, only to find she was blue, not breathing, and on the floor in the midst of a heart attack. She was rushed to the hospital and placed in surgery where her heart kept stopping. Apparently, it took them hours to get the heart beating regularly and required a heart pacemaker. Dad didn't mention that my phone call probably saved Mom's life, but I knew.

Mom had another miracle happen years later. Of course, the doctors didn't think so, but I knew again. She developed one of the worst forms of cancer, of the pancreas—a cancer for which there was no cure or even good treatment, especially since by the time a person has symptoms, it is already stage 4 metastatic. The average survival from point of diagnosis at the time was three months—something I learned while visiting a scientist at the NIH when I walked over to see the top cancer scientist at the National Cancer Institute—Mom's records in hand. He sadly told me they didn't even have experimental drugs that showed hope.

I had been praying for my parents for some time after becoming a believer myself, and when she got that lethal cancer, my prayers were for her complete healing since only a miracle of God would save her. I got a letter (back when letters and not email were the norm) from Mom telling me about her visit to a church to listen to a singing student of hers (Mom and Dad never went to church, other than the CE—Christmas/Easter versions—to show business friends they were not anti-religious and for business promotions, I guessed). Mom said she never felt so loved in a church before and might like to go back. It was that unusual, spirit-filled Mexican American church, that had services in Spanish (her first language, living with my grandfather as a missionary to South America).

My upcoming visit included going with her to this special church where she felt that special love. Mom was so weak with her cancer that I had to walk with her and hold her up some, but she came. She was tough. Amazingly, they had a visiting evangelist speaking that day, who was called to pray for healing of others. Halfway through the service, Mom didn't think she could last and asked if we could go. Not wanting to miss out on his prayers, I sent word to the pastor to see if we could get a prayer session before we left, and it was set up in a back room. Then the visiting evangelist—an overly young guy with the West Virginia kind of Southern drawl—did something I had never seen. He breathed (actually blowed) at her and said, "receive the spirit of God" or something similar (I later learned that the same words used for the Holy Spirit were "breath of God"). When he laid his hands on Mom and blowed on her, she began to weep. I had never seen my mom weep before, so I did too.

Leaving the church that day, mom told me something happened to her in there. I responded in my knowing way—"yes, you were touched by God" or "the Holy Spirit was in the room." But she said, "No, something happened to me there. Something *came into me*." Wow, did God really come into her that day, I wondered? The next morning, I left and will never forget the way she looked at me from the driveway. I think there were streams of white light coming from her eyes. Her cancer went away. We would say there was some kind of spontaneous remission, but I didn't buy it. There was nothing spontaneous about it, I concluded. Mom lived a year after that—long after she was supposed to have died from her adenocarcinoma of the pancreas—and the cancer came back with a vengeance. That was a special year for Mom and Dad, who traveled around the country and did things she always wanted to do.

In between the time of my seemingly "coincidental" Mom lifesaving call and her "spontaneous" healing from cancer, the hounds caught up with me big time. I was broken, frozen, and ready for breakthrough. A couple days after reluctantly entering the halfway house, marriage-less and heart wounded, I decided to go back to visit the church in which we were married. It was probably just to get out of the house on a pass, since church attendance was not only allowed, but encouraged. I recall asking about the spiritual "part" of the AA 12-Step program and was severely corrected: "There is no spiritual part of the 12-Step program, it *is* a spiritual program!" My sponsors would roundly agree.

Brokenhearted and in such emotional pain, I strangely went up at the end of the service for prayer. I wanted the pastor to pray to bring my wife back. The prayer he prayed seemed to be just what I wanted: "Lord, please give John a *new* relationship." I was satisfied. If God was there and had heard this spiritual prayer, then he would bring her back. It wasn't long before I came to know this was Christian code for a relationship with Christ Jesus. It had nothing to do with getting my wife back. In fact, it was just the opposite.

God now had two deals in the "bank." I contracted to give my life to Him, *and now* was bound to have a new relationship—*with him*. The hounds chased me up that tree and soon leapt on me when I fell out of the tree after the (last) limb I was hanging on broke.

Suicide Flight

It was two days later, in excruciating heart pain, that I died. It was a leap of hope where it didn't matter to me whether I lived or died.

I'm not sure how many people can relate to such a state or decision, but it was like standing on a ledge or mountain rock face and just letting go—falling forward to whatever destiny lay below. I was either going to be caught and saved or would perish. Either way would be okay, to end the pain. The prayer (my third, I guess) was the most powerful of all!

I was sitting in my car behind the VA hospital where I worked—just after my noontime AA meeting, one of my favorites. I had stopped drinking some months earlier, but still attended for support and my new "church." It was more of a desperate demand rather than a sweet prayer we often hear about. I had had it with this life and misery, and while I was not going to kill myself, actively that is, I no longer cared if I did die. In a way I did: "God, if you are there, I need to know NOW! I need to feel your power NOW!" That was the exact prayer. I remember it well, because of what happened next.

Letting go completely, it was like falling and waiting to hit bottom. The rocks. This was strange since I was always afraid of heights and the last thing I would ever do was get close to a precipice or ledge, much less let go and fall. But I did that in my mind, and the experience was much like giving up and letting go, falling, with little hope of being saved. The cliff image and the falling over the edge represented my surrender. People who have experienced this sort of profound surrender, especially of the spiritual kind, know what I'm talking about. Something took over. It was like I was caught in God's hands. I believe and later learned of a Bible scripture representing what I had done: "If you seek Me with all your heart, you will truly find Me" (Jeremiah 29:13). And I did, I guess, His hands, His love.

My sense of control over my emotions and physical feelings was gone, no longer under my volition. A warm, liquid substance felt like it was seeping, or welling up, inside me and spreading around my body, from gut to chest to arms and head. Then a kind of joyful giggle welled up inside me, strangely because I was not a joyful giggler and in no place to do such craziness, and I felt the most wonderful love filling me from the inside and out. The experience lasted for about 20 minutes, and I had visions that I will detail more in another (hoped for) book. But my life changed in that altered state.

I remember while this was happening and taking over, thinking with what residual control I had left, this must be what it is like to go crazy—to have a psychotic break. But this was completely different than what I had experienced on LSD. That was terror, this was liquid joy and a welcome and needed loss of old control. There was peace in this "break from reality," not horror with bloody fire-breathing serpent-like visions. If I ever come back to reality, I thought, I will have to tell my students and colleagues in psychology what it was like. But I never came back to that reality. After that, my life was a series of attempts to find out what had happened, pursue God and truth, get out of psychology, or alternatively find a way to integrate what had happened into my practice of psychology. It would become the latter, The Integration.

So, I attempted to "integrate" my developing faith walk with my profession, and I found creative ways to attempt it. I connected with churches, especially African American churches and foreign ministries, and worked with HIV/AIDS in Africa, even adding an intercessory prayer component to a large study on treatment of recovering alcoholic smokers. Crazy. Let me tell you about all that in the coming chapter—the crossroads of my faith and my profession—a potential train wreck, or a wonderful merging and marriage. Guess.

ROOM 602

SPIRITUAL INTEGRATION CROSSROADS

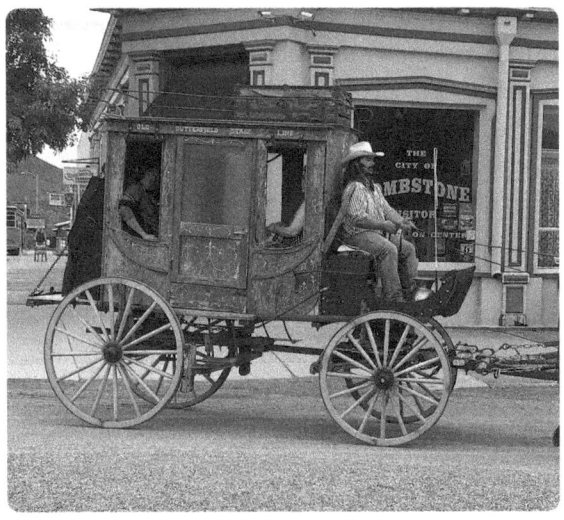

*"Don't look back.
You're not going that way."*

—UNKNOWN

The Crossroads

The AA *Big Book* describes coming to a "crossroads" or turning point, in one's road to recovery, and I had as well. A wooden stake was driven between my career and life as a psychologist, professor, and researcher and some sort of a transformative spiritual awakening, a "new life." Some said I was "born again," but I wasn't so sure what had happened to me. I figured I had either gone crazy, as I've said, or it had to do with God. "Where do I go from here?" I wondered, "Stay in psychology or leave somehow, and for what, and to where?" Pretty big questions.

What would you do? Become a religious nut and go off the deep end, as some (former) friends and associates warned, or just figure it was merely a "phase" that would pass—as my former mentor suggested—and stay the course? Should I wait for my "heart attack" to subside, heal if need be, and get back to regular business, as (ab)normal? Or should I go the other, new direction in life. To say that it was a critical decision would be the proverbial understatement. I considered pulling up all those professional tent stakes tying me down and going rogue and radical, like my Ivy League (Dartmouth) grandfather who walked away from a career in engineering to become a missionary, pastor, and minister of the Gospel. My mother did say I was a lot (maybe too much) like him.

It was ironic that one of my prayers in supposedly turning my life over to God and His direction was: "God, I will do anything for you and go anywhere you lead, but just *not* to Africa!" Where did that come from? Anyway, I had never heard the scriptural quip, "If you want to make God laugh, tell Him your plans." In my case, what were *not* my plans, what I was *not* going to do. Indeed, John plans, God laughs, as He must have done with my prayer. But wouldn't you know, Africa, here I come (but not yet). It was a creative (and maybe humorous, God humor that is) feat how He got me there.

I remember a conversation with my mother in our kitchen one day during my spiritual transformation journey. I was trying to explain how I found her father's, my grandfather's, Bible he preached out of—with all the notes and commentary revealing his heart for God, how precious that was to me. Strangely to me, it seemed to terrify her, as I heard the unlikely, fear-filled demand—"You're not becoming one of those Jesus freaks, are you?!"

I thought for a long moment as we stood face-to-face in silent contention. Rather than taking offense at the argument bait, I responded with love and grace. Where did *that* come from? Not her firebrand son, John. Certainly not me. But I think maybe God's Spirit gave me the words that followed: "Mom, I don't know what

I'm becoming, but I sure like the direction." We stood silently, face-to-face, for what seemed like a long time in new understanding—probably more like 30 seconds. Looking back now on our kitchen conversation that day, I think fondly of my mom with her loving fearfulness for her "favorite" father-like (favorite) son, and I decided to never forget.

Initially, I tried to get the heck out of psychology after this bombastic, psychotic-like spiritual "awakening" of mine. But God had other plans for me it seemed, and what did I know. From that perspective, I was worshipping at the wrong altar—humanistic philosophies and secularized science that began with the frankly unscientific, a priori conclusion that there was no God—but then I rationalized it certainly didn't mean I had to *leave* psychology *entirely*. Maybe I could redefine it, make a compromise between the two tug-of-war sides—create a new career focus or direction. Some in the Christian world, especially academics like myself, call it "integration." But it was oil and water. How do they, or can they even, combine or integrate?

A part of me was averse to change, but I had been changed. Nevertheless, I had devoted so much to psychology, becoming a clinical psychologist and struggling up the academic and research ladders of success (I still believed Dad would have been proud of me, though he never said it). It was a lot to give up, and I didn't know if I could. Then what would I do? Trust God completely? Phew. I just wasn't there, though I was close. It depended on the day. But then God and a few strategic others stepped in to help resolve this great divide, the conflict between the old me, all I had accomplished to get where I was (wherever that was, I now wondered!), and the newborn me. I'd been cut loose, hanging by a finger, and despite it all I was held. As I call it to mind now, I can't help but think of God's outstretched hand reaching toward Adam in Michelangelo's mural adorning the Sistine Chapel.

I remember a (more mature) "undercover" Christian colleague at the medical school advising me when I privately shared my dilemma. She encouraged me in a different way than I expected or hoped:

"Maybe God wants to use you *in* the field, not *out* of it. Don't leave; see what He does with you and it." That made strange but useful sense, so eventually I decided to stay and pursue both. Dr. John, the "integrationist"! Yeah, right. There were many times I thought I made the wrong decision, bypassing that path of radicalness for and in God and the other side of fame and achievement in psychology. Ego versus spirit, pressing on in my psychological life and making (spiritual) lemonade along the way—to integrate my new faith and hope with my career. It was an interesting, creative adventure and rocky road, to be sure.

Finally, deciding I could serve both God and my field of psychology, together as much as possible—a great integration of faith and profession—I embarked on that quest at first awkwardly, like a toddler learning to walk with new leg. I think it was the Apostle Paul who said he was a "fool for Christ"—good company indeed. Remember my work with precious Michael at the children's hospital, who had that condition that made his legs unusable from birth? They were later amputated so he could be fitted with little starter prosthetic legs, and then full-sized ones as he grew. He needed crutches for quite some time to learn to walk on them. That was me too: new spiritual legs, old ones removed, learning to walk a new walk.

Bringing the Mountain to Moses
I decided earlier on in my faith integration quest that if the church wouldn't come to me at the university, then I would go to it. I sought connection with churches, especially African American churches, for my clinical intervention research locally, and then foreign ministries and work with HIV/AIDS in Africa. As I mentioned earlier, I even added an intercessory prayer component to a large study on treatment of recovering alcoholic smokers, but I'm getting ahead of myself in this story.

I recalled the conversation with a more well-known colleague who threatened my fast-rising career with this religious stuff (he probably used a different adjective, but we will stick with "stuff"). He was not alone, as I came to find out. I remember a doorway conversation with a member of the tenure and promotion committee who had participated in denying my tenure (later rescinded by the dean and the higher-ups). My new faith, not so hidden at first, was a threat to the otherwise religious as well as the anti-religious. I was different, and certainly unwise in not keeping this to myself. But how could I? It was gushing out of me (I later learned of one of my favorite Bible scriptures in John 7:38, that described it well). Like when my mom called me a Jesus freak, and my dad called me a bigot. It was hard to hear even though I understood their fear and *protective* judgments.

I figured I'd go out in flames! What did I have to lose? I tried to do so in various ways beginning with my heading west, to California, out of the proverbial Bible Belt and into the land of "spiritual darkness." God didn't go west of Arizona, I half joked with friends. (I learned later about the powerful Jesus movement, with amazing new worship music by saved rock stars—including Bob Dylan, later—that occurred during the '60s and '70s in Southern California.)

I was still too hardheaded and arrogant to get faith and belief the way more humble people do—who just hear, decide, and believe. That wasn't me. I was the "puffed up with knowledge and without wisdom" kind who required a mind-blowing miraculous blast to see and be transformed beyond my control. The groundwork for my personal and spiritual transformation started, not surprisingly, with stopping drinking (finding a "new spirit"), becoming as some say a "12-Step Christian," attending as many meetings as I could at my new AA "church," learning to pray and reading the Bible, and seeking and creating opportunities for integrating that faith and belief—you might say surgically implanting it—in my research and teaching at the university. What fun!

"Your career will be ruined," that well-known colleague warned me, should I try to impose my new religious spirituality (called pejoratively "religiosity" by many) on my career and other unsuspecting psychology people. So, to the flames it was, with some trepidation but also with a spice of crazy faith. Others even on my conference committee were wary, and clearly distanced themselves from me, their "religious nut" former friend and close colleague.

I was torn even between my successful and growing career as a professor and researcher, and my new spiritual and religious path. It meant that in many cases my friends were not going to be as close as before, and that hurt. But it was one of those good pains, or hurts.

The year of my spiritual upheaval, I happened to be the chair of my behavior therapy association's international convention in Philadelphia, 1984. This was a time when it was still not okay in my field to talk about spirituality, God especially. So when I decided to put together a symposium titled: "Integrating Behavioral and Spiritual Approaches to Change"[22], the die was cast on my career ruination. I had to tell my review committee that this one would not go through review. I was inserting it in the convention. I asked several well-known colleagues in the behavior therapy field to participate. They had written on the topic of spirituality and behavior change, and each accepted with enthusiasm. Despite the fact that the symposium was on the last afternoon of the whole convention—the death knell for most any talk since attendees would usually leave to fly back home—it was standing room only.

The audience of behavior therapists covered the gamut of spiritual and religious backgrounds and interests, and with their encouragement my colleague and friend who helped set it up, Bill Miller, created a special interest group and newsletter on this topic. An edited book by the two of us followed. The ink on my demise from psychology, and especially behavior therapy, was cast deeper still, and my career was now on the fast track to destruction. But not quite.

Around this time, following my spiritual and religious transition, word got out through my former resident, Charlie Carlson, who did a Bible study with me in my office, and I began to be invited to churches and one well-known Christian college—Wheaton College—where one of Charlie's fellow psychology interns at my program was the head of the psychology department. That might have been a direction for me to pursue, teaching at a Christian college or university, but I was very new in my faith journey, and had much to process and integrate with my profession. I just didn't feel the release from God to essentially abandon all that I had achieved and accomplished for a very different professional life.

Then another thing happened—a great new job offer that I became convinced God was in—and I was drawn elsewhere, still in the secular university and medical school setting. Anyway, as it turned out, years later I did toss my hat into that arena, and even then, it wasn't for me (or for God with me, apparently).

When they brought me up to Chicago to give a talk at Wheaton, the introduction Stan gave me was short and remarkable, but not very "sweet": "I want to introduce someone who was the least likely person to ever become a Christian, Dr. John Martin." Oh boy, I didn't expect that kind of a testimonial. I wasn't sure how to react. Was I that bad? Truth be told, yes, I was. I took it the best way: nothing is too hard for God to do, and I was in his sights (probably due to the many who had been praying for me, unbeknownst to me).

I could not remain underground for long and found myself attracted to Christian schools and churches for talks and training, especially in South Africa, where I had done two teaching sabbaticals, and South Korea, at a seminary that was connected to my faculty position at a seminary in Pasadena (where there were many Korean students).

Marriage Therapist?
In my earlier attempts to integrate, and possibly revitalize my clinical practice, I decided to be completely transparent about my past, such as my marriage failures. So I confessed to couples interested in marriage counseling that I would probably not be the psychologist to help them as I had never been successful at marriage, but that I would help evaluate and refer them to a competent, healing therapist. Would you believe they would call me back after my first and only planned session with them and (typically the wife) tell me they (the husband especially) definitely wanted to work with me! I think the husband probably told the wife something like, "he has been through marriage struggles and will understand me better." I stopped telling couples that after this happened a number of times (with me trying to fire myself after that first session), and the husband wanting *me*. Okay, I got it.

Road to the "Dark Side"—California

Not long after, and waiting for the other career shoe to drop, I ended up on a short list of applicants for a new position out West, directing a doctoral program in my field of behavioral medicine and health psychology. My mentor and doctoral thesis advisor was the number one candidate and was ready to accept the position. Number two was another colleague, much more advanced and qualified than I. I was number three. Number one apparently accepted the position, but at the last minute changed his mind and withdrew, while I understood that number two was not happy about not being selected as number one, and he withdrew as well—leaving almost completely unqualified me.

Knowing it was not God who was leading me West (remember, God did not go west of Arizona), I decided to be sure, and I agreed to interview. Then came the interesting part. As usual, I got to meet the higher-ups, deans, department chairs, and some prominent researchers, as well as give presentations at the university and medical schools, which would be hiring me for this joint appointment. It was a job clearly over my head, especially since I had never administrated such a large program—only smaller research grant programs.

It was conspiracy theory time! I knew how I would confirm this was not of God. I spoke, foolishly if not stupidly, in every interview and meeting with these deans and directors regarding my faith—how I could no longer separate my faith and belief in God, and my Christian walk, from my academic and research life and career, including in this new position should I be offered it. This, as you might guess, is academic suicide. You *never* confess such a thing, much less reveal you will include your religious spirituality in what you plan to do at the university or medical school. I unknowingly and wrongly assumed that medical school and medical sciences would be the least open to a faith-driven professor and researcher. In fact, it was the other way around, I eventually found out. The university setting and especially psychology departments there were among the least religious- or faith-tolerant places. I clearly identified myself as that token Jesus freak, that they should not want anything to do with, much less hire for their highly secular position. But, God laughing almost audibly, my plan didn't work.

My first presentation at the medical school went pretty well, but it was the second one, on my return interview visit to the university side, that did not. Apparently, the message was left on my phone machine that I would need to give a second talk before the university on the upcoming interview. I never got it. It was at dinner, the night before the planned but unknown presentation, that I was asked what I would be presenting on, and my response was perfect: "Presentation? What presentation?" I think my friend and colleague Bob, who was part of the recruiting team there at the school, went pale. So, there I was without even a single slide or talk preparation, and I was up the next day. What to do?

I prayed and gave it to God. "Okay, God, if this job is for me, and I believe it is not for me or of You, you will have to figure this out." I even asked to take about five minutes, go behind the curtain separating the stage from the large audience of faculty and students "breathlessly" awaiting a great talk, and pray. I embarked without any audiovisuals on a journey through my research studies, stories from one question and findings to another in as simple a fashion as I could put together. It seemed to work, amazingly, and I received compliments on how well it went.

At this point, I knew I would not (and should not) get the job offer, and then would be on my way back to my old job, which I liked very much, at the VA and medical center. Simplicity, peace. Crisis averted. Problem solved.

But the folks out West didn't cooperate. I was offered the position. *Now* what to do? The offer was very attractive and with nice salary and benefits, so I told them I needed to think and pray (I actually said that) about it. I should say that I was taken aback at how beautiful it was there in California, next to the Pacific Ocean, and with such an exciting new position that I could grow into.

A further wrinkle in my resolve that this was not God (but the other one, the tempter) was that in their first doctoral class, two of the ten students were born-again Christians. Knowing some about my faith, they asked me if I would like to attend church with them while out there on interview, and I accepted. Early that Sunday morning, before church, I think God woke me up and spoke silently to my heart, kind of like telling me He was in this. You may know about hearing God's voice—the still small voice that you hear in your heart and mind, not audibly, but nevertheless understandably. Further, sitting down in church when the choir began their worship, I broke down into silent weeping—throughout the whole service! How embarrassing, I thought. I felt that still small voice again, informing me that I needed to start letting go of my old job.

So, I headed back east with a lot on my mind and heart. I didn't know what to do. Where was God in this? I continued to try to convince myself that I was not supposed to head West and take that job, but I needed more confirmation of that. I think my closest colleagues on the recruitment committee knew I was praying about the position and offer, and they respected it. I was grateful to them, especially my colleagues Bob and Al. Then I came up with a "foolproof" (for fool John) way to know and get confirmation. I did something I never had done—I "acted as if" every other day. On one day, I envisioned and acted as if I was taking the job and leaving to go West. I focused my thoughts and imagination as if I was going, and already there. What would it be like there? What would it be like leaving my job and friends? Then, the following day, I switched it. I imagined and envisioned that I turned down the offer and was staying. What would it be like knowing I said no to the new opportunity, and was staying put? This went on, day after day, for two weeks.

I remember the day that friends approached me and expressed concerns that I seemed depressed or down. It was the day I was going to stay in my present job and turn down the California position. They also noted the opposite, on those days dedicated to deciding to accept the position and head for California—on those days, I seemed much happier, one of them even noticing a light coming from my eyes.

I told no one about this plan, so they were all unaware. It was, in effect, a single-blind study (in some ways, it was double-blind since I was not aware of how I was acting and feeling until the very end).

The light and passion for California then began to grow—irrepressibly despite my resistance to leaving—and I had finally decided, or it had been decided for me. I called them, accepted the position, and began my preparations for leaving and saying goodbye to my friends, church, colleagues, and even my new Christian girlfriend, Becky. My current affiliations made a very good counteroffer, but I had decided. So it was off to California and the new position for which I had absolutely *no* background or experience.

It was a crazy transition, especially since I was leaving my girlfriend, with no guarantee we would go on to get married (which we ultimately did), and the job was brand new and overwhelming to this relatively young (late 30s) professor. A distinguished colleague and editor of a book I helped write gave me a prophetic congratulations. When hearing of my accepting the job, he said: "Congratulations, and condolences" (i.e., your research career is over). I think the latter was said with different words but carried the same meaning—and he was nearly right. Nevertheless, it was not only a whole new career in some ways—teaching undergrad and graduate students, directing a large and distinguished new joint doctoral program that combined my two areas of behavioral medicine and psychological research and training—it was California. You know, sun, ocean, and sailing! And I was certain that it was God. I was being led there, for better or worse.

There was a "new guard" of friends and colleagues who wanted me there, helped recruit me, and then became my weekly running buddies at our beach jog together that lasted for years. Then there was the "old guard" of professors who had been in the large university department (45 Ph.D. professors) who were not so excited about my joining the faculty and co-leading this new joint doctoral program between the university school of psychology and psychiatry at the medical school—to compete with the major California psychology and psychiatry training programs.

Some were downright against me being there and sought from the beginning to try to get rid of me. I wasn't tenured on the way in but had been promised it by the dean within a year—which I just barely squeaked in, thanks to the dean and all the way up to the academic

VP of the school overruling the department's promotion committee's denial of my tenure. I was ready to leave given that vote of "no confidence" but, need I say, that was apparently not God's plan.

Seeking Spiritual Integration: Taking Research to the Church
A most interesting new program was my work testing exercise in the treatment of high blood pressure. In my Project HELPS (Hypertension Exercise Lifestyle Program for Seniors), a large NIH-funded project, we noticed that we had very few African Americans enrolled in the project. This was concerning because blacks have two to three times the risk of high blood pressure and heart disease than non-blacks, so all the more reason for having a decent population sample in our project.

Checking with other researchers at my university, I was asked why I didn't go to the Ministerial Alliance, the African American and Hispanic coalition headed by pastors and priests and minority community leaders. So, I approached them and asked for a meeting. When the meeting day came up, I went in, unbeknownst, as a sacrificial lamb. While in the meeting room, I was surrounded by distinguished minority leaders and subjected to a heated lecture about Tuskegee Study—the horrible abuse against African Americans. That was the years-ago medical study out of Tuskegee, Alabama, that followed black men who were suffering with syphilis, including being denied very promising experimental antibiotic treatments, so as to determine the disease progression. It was a horrible, pre-ethics–committee, and pre-civil–rights example of a highly unethical study that did or allowed harm to its participants.

I think the sweat coming down my face was observable to all, and I was imagining how quick I could exit from the room. They concluded that they were sick and tired as a community of having researchers and professors like myself coming down from the ivory tower on high, using their community, and leaving, with no benefit ever to them. Finally stopping, they looked at me for my response. I was panicked, but something came over me, and I decided, humbly, to not only take the well-deserved verbal whipping, but to make fun of myself. So I said: "Does anyone possibly have a blood pressure cuff? I think my blood pressure has gone way up!" Almost surprising to me, this comment broke the tension and ice in the room, and they all laughed that gut- level laugh, and I laughed with them. My feet had been held to the fire, I'd been tested, and then accepted. They decided this uppity professor was all right, and apparently someone they would be willing to work with.

This led to my invite into both the Jackie Robinson YMCA community and one of the large full gospel black churches there. I actually moved part of my program to that church and worked closely with the Y on cardiovascular health and smoking treatment, where I would bring my teams of students and research assistants.

One project I devised with the help of the minority community was to address a significant problem in black Americans—prostate cancer. Younger black men have roughly three times the risk of contracting and dying from (especially undiagnosed) prostate cancer. It was not an easy thing to get any man to submit himself to the awful digital prostate exam, which at the time was the best way to determine cancerous growths on that male organ. I decided to ask them, scheduling a focus group. I went around to churches and community meetings to recruit black men, offering free movie tickets and Hometown Buffet meals for just showing up and talking with me.

The day for the focus group meeting arrived, and I showed up at the full gospel church with a student helper, and you know how many showed up? Zero. I couldn't figure out what I had done wrong or neglected. That was until I was taken aside by one of the senior ladies from the church and told: "Honey, you're never going to ever get our black husbands, brothers, and sons to come to a health meeting. You talked to the wrong people. You should have been talking to us ladies. We are the ones in charge of our men and boys' health."

This was another "NOW you tell me." Unfortunately, as goes many a creative and important research project, we never were able to resurrect the study and intervention, though I'm not sure why. I think other issues and projects elbowed their way into my research and clinical path, I decided to work more directly with the African

American church and their health issues, and there was the issue of funding for the new project of prostate cancer. I had gotten overextended, something none of my colleagues ever did. Yeah, right.

Travels to Africa (Prayer Denied!)
I was invited for two teaching sabbaticals in South Africa in 1994 and then in 2001.

I found to my pleasant surprise that English was their default language out of the eight native and Afrikaner languages *and* that it was a strongly Christian nation. Many have said that it was their Christian churches, their faith, and much prayer, that led to their bloodless revolution and free election, more than anything else. My new faith fit in well with their strong Christian heritage and practice, including university church life. My love for the country and people led to seven more trips there on both teaching and research, as well as for Christian mission work in the townships and historically black colleges and universities. In Africa, I was no longer a spiritual "fish out of water" as I was in the US.

The team I had joined in Uganda for a two-week training seminar I helped teach was from the United Kingdom, and I was apparently the only Christian or churchgoing member. This caused some concern for them—until, that is, the nurses requested that I talk about spiritual approaches to helping people change—right up my new alley! So, with the team leader's reluctant approval, I spent a whole afternoon talking about spiritual approaches to motivation and God's science of change. It was a wonderful opportunity to integrate my faith with my practice as a professor of psychology and clinician.

Another opportunity of mine, dropped in my lap (by God?) was in, of all places, Eastern Germany—the atheist, communist-controlled area within the Soviet Union before the wall fell. I was on teaching sabbatical there, and before I began, I was asked if I could teach on Christian psychology—a topic I had written on and included in my CV. I was already tenured at this point and considered the token fundamentalist "Jesus freak." The damage to my career had already been done, if any, and I was freed from concerns over that anymore.

Isn't that what tenure is about? I was told yes, but there was an exception for religious nuts, who were not covered.

I was so excited about this request I would have *paid* them to let me teach it—though I didn't confess this, as I accepted their payment for this teaching as well. I found that the very interested students knew little to nothing about the Bible or Christianity, so I had to lay the foundation by teaching some from the Bible before discussing what became known as "Christian psychology"—something I kind of thought was a contradiction in terms! It was an actual thing! I guess I was a Christian psychologist, not just a Christian who happened to be a psychologist.

> **CAN WE TALK?**
>
> *Christian Psychology vs. Secular Psychology.* I struggled for a while with what I was—a Christian who taught and did psychology, or a Christian psychologist who practiced the Christian (Biblical?) version of psychology. I graduated to the latter for the most part, but never presented myself as that exclusively. I worked with, did therapy with, and taught and conducted research on all kinds of people, of all faiths and creeds, and I never pushed my faith on any. I do remember walking out on a so-called Christian therapist who never prayed with my wife and me, even when I asked. She was a psychologist who was (secondarily) a Christian. I found a number like that, students and faculty alike (of all places) at the seminary.
>
> *Suggestion:* If you are looking for a psychologist of strong, primarily Christian faith and practice, then ask him or her how they see psychology and what place it has in relation to the Bible, the church, and Christian faith and practice. Don't assume. I've seen too many people and couples who have gotten "stuck" with a psychologist or therapist who happened to be a Christian, by name but not practice, and failed to represent their or the Bible's Christianity. It can be a big gulf between the two, but there is no necessary contradiction between evidence-based psychology and Christian faith and practice. A great example of this is the field and style

> of motivational interviewing and counseling[5], which successfully integrates motivation science, spiritual, and biblical truths (e.g., "agape" love) approaches to helping people change[23]. The 12-Step programs are spiritual programs with a strong Christian core, and many churches now have Christian and Bible-based 12-Step programs, such as Celebrate Recovery (CR) developed by Rick Warren's Saddleback Church. There is a large clinical and research literature devoted to Christian psychology, and I encourage interested readers to investigate it.

And then there were the spiritual therapies of which I became a student and professor. I connected with two students more closely, whom I brought over to the US on an internship paid by their school, to attend my teaching and participate in my research. They also attended church and Christian fellowships with me as well, and I believe both had spiritual transformations while in the US with me.

Pastoral Training and Practice
Some time after my trip to Africa, I (or God, who knows?) decided it was time to get more formal training as a Christian, to become a pastor, in both my community volunteer work and in my clinical practice. I enrolled in a two-year school of ministry at my large evangelical church, and at about the same time helped to develop and implement their new Christian 12-Step program—Celebrate Recovery (CR)—with my good friend, Bible study bicycle ride buddy, and future best man at my marriage, Steve Henning.

I became a much more serious student of the Bible after that, and as a part of my internship there in the church's ministry school, I was plugged into the ministries for seniors at nursing homes and facilities for the elderly and developed a real love for those often lonely and frequently disabled ones. When I was offered a chance to lead a Bible study and worship program for a large shelter for the mentally disabled, I jumped at it (it made sense, a psychologist there), and I continue to lead to this day. I was even married there, in a joy-filled, *One Flew Over the Cuckoo's Nest* (with the Holy Spirit!) ceremony before God, attended by our friends and all the residents at the shelter home, whom we loved and who loved us so much.

I was still commuting weekly to my university when an opportunity to move to an actual Christian doctoral training program at a well-known theological seminary arose, and I was invited to apply. I decided to and was offered a position as tenured professor of clinical psychology, which after much prayer and counsel from close friends, I accepted.

It was not my best decision as it turned out, leaving a much bigger university and department where I was spoiled, getting to teach only the courses I wanted to and that were in my specialty areas. Not so in the new, small department where everyone had to teach pretty much every course. My time there was eventful, both positive and not so positive, as I was more a fish out of water as a charismatic ("Jesus freak"), newer, wet-behind-the-theological-ears Christian. We all pretty much came to realize the fit was not that good on either end. Shortly thereafter, with some encouragement from the higher-ups (and God, it turned out), I volunteered to leave after three short years. It didn't help that I was going through a breakup and depression over a failing relationship (prior to my years-later marriage to my beautiful wife, Catherine).

One memorable occasion while there at the seminary caused a jaw-dropping reaction from me. I was giving clinical therapy supervision to advanced doctoral students when I asked how with Christian clients, they introduced and practiced prayer along with their evidence-based psychological therapies (many were interning at Christian churches and therapy centers). The students were shocked at my question. They declared that would be "unethical." WHAT? My shocked response—how ethical would it be to fail (or refuse) to include prayer to God, the Helper, Great Physician, and Wonderful Counselor, who could completely heal the client or work in combination with their practice of evidence-based psychological and behavioral counseling? A formal complaint against me was registered with the associate dean over this episode as far as I knew. This and other issues, such as my sometimes not-so-great teaching evaluations, led to three meetings to decide on my fate.

Besides the apparently exclusionary emphasis on the methods of secular psychology over the true integration of biblical and Holy Spirit approaches to counseling and therapy, there were some other difficulties I had with my school's approach and teachings. There were exceptions to this criticism, especially my friend and colleague Siang-Yang Tan and some others who believed and taught integration the way I thought was right, while being careful not to place psychology on a pedestal above God, the Holy Spirit, and biblical truth. It was an occupational hazard.

I was also concerned (along with the school, to be honest) with the great cost of the doctoral training at that private institution, reaching a quarter-million dollars for some in their five-to-six-year program. This was especially problematic given the fact that many graduates, deeply in debt, had significant problems finding jobs, particularly those that could permit repayment of their loans. My school was not alone in struggling with this problem.

All things considered, especially my bad fit for them, I offered my lifetime tenured professorship back to the school (are you *crazy*, John? Yes) and walked away into life as a licensed clinical psychologist and therapist. Once again, a "now what" time, as I stepped down to the clinical trenches of therapy with individuals and couples—a much better fit for this semiretired psychology professor. I was happier too.

Because of my Christian background and interests shown on my internet bios at places such as *Psychology Today* (the big source for people finding a suitable therapist), I began to attract many Christians and Christian couples to my practice. Concluding I needed all the help I could get in working with these oftentimes complex and chronic problems in relationships and personal functioning, especially communication, forgiveness, addictions, anxiety and depression, trauma, and PTSD, I tried to include prayer to begin and end sessions. Some clients guessed that it was God's intervention and Spirit in the sessions much more than my work that made the positive difference. They were right!

I also got involved in two wonderful helping ministries that addressed psychological and relationship issues—Celebrate Recovery (CR) a 12-Step type of program for the addictions, including sexual addiction developed and expanded to many churches by Rick Warren and Saddleback Church (celebraterecovery.com), and New Life Ministries a powerful and effective Christian-based program led by Steve Arterburn (newlife.com), which conducted various weekend workshops for couples and individuals. Along with Barnabas, I was able to help lead small groups through New Life (especially their "Every Man's Battle" for men with sexual addiction) and to help set up and lead the CR program at my church. These were wonderful places for me to integrate my newfound faith with my field of psychology—but with a Christian perspective and approach.

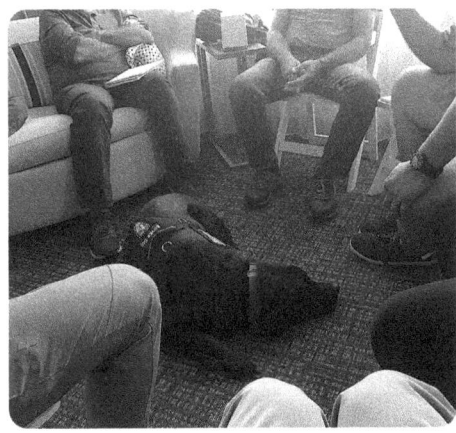

Integrating Motivation, Science, and Faith

As part of my own integration of faith and psychology, I found that motivational interviewing and counseling was a great fit. Being a newer student, adherent, and then teacher/trainer of the motivational style of helping people change, it was natural to think about adapting this approach to the church and her ministries. This connection seemed especially appropriate since motivational interviewing, the applied version of motivation science, was consistent with spiritual principles of freedom and autonomy, nonjudgmental or directing gentle guidance (not programming), and respect for individual choice, readiness, and personal ability. My top master's student, Scott Walters, who went on to a distinguished career as a professor of psychology and public health, told me about a motivational approach to his teaching a Sunday school class. I liked it, so I integrated it into my work with churches and faith-based schools and groups.

Using the values clarification exercise, as with the female client who wanted a family, he added God's values to the discussion—picked out by the students. For example, for the values clarification exercise, clients would be asked to first rate and order their personal top values, what is most important in their lives, perhaps picking their leading 10 values. Then a motivational dialogue takes place when clients are asked to compare some issue in their lives—like drinking, drug use, anger, failing to seek a new job or relationship with desirable people (as with our female client)—with the individual values they had chosen, such as happiness, health, family, love, success, and so on. Their rating would indicate whether the issue helped, hurt, or had no effect on supporting, enhancing, or achieving the value.

But Scott added *God's values* for the individual, not just their own. In this case, the Bible study or church students would conduct a comparison of their own values with God's values for them (for example, from the Bible) and behaviors (such as premarital sex, drug, and alcohol use, etc.). Then they would have their motivational dialogue and collaboration, comparing their values comparison results with those of God's values for them. It was such a great idea that I stole it from Scott and have used it since in my training in churches and seminaries in Africa and Korea, with my seminary doctoral student, Priscilla E. P. Sihn. Thank you, Scott.

My attempt to integrate my newer faith with my profession as a psychologist and professor ventured the international road, from Korea teaching motivational interviewing at the seminary there to Romania, where I conducted that motivational counseling debate at the high school described in the previous chapter on my world traveling professoring. Romania was that mission trip where I talked about my fun time with the crazed students looking to destroy me in my "losing" argument over drugs, alcohol, and sex. Admittedly, Romania was more a secular than a spiritual integration, but the approach has a strong spiritual core or foundation, in which one can talk about the *spirit* of effective counseling. I call it effective, strategic, spiritual, and behavioral change evocation—being "quick to listen and slow to speak" and ready to encourage and love kind of reflective motivational counseling. I made that last part up but it sounds good anyway.

Ask the Professor
Another fun effort at faith integration happened on the street!—consisting of my "Ask the Professor" (ATP) crazy "motivational" evangelism. I would put on my three-striped doctoral gown and cap, with school colors on the hood, and head for the beach near where I live. I would post a large sign: "Ask the Professor," sometimes using the flip side "Stump the Professor," and wait for suspecting souls to come have a dialogue. Most wouldn't know what to ask, so I would hand them a list of possible questions, including why I was out there making a fool of myself and then things like, "What do you have faith in?" "Is the Bible true?" "How do you get to heaven?" "Is personality testing accurate?" and so on. I'd often bring a friend to help, and sometimes we would blow huge bubbles (you've seen those) to draw a crowd—or at least kids and their parents. I've gotten into some beautiful conversations and would practice my motivational counseling, listening, and reflecting to engage their most interesting questions and open dialogue.

I remember some of the conversations I had with passersby curious about what in the world I was doing out there by the pier gowned up next to my ASK sign. There were four types of folks who approached me.

First ATP-ers were the believers. These were curious about whether I was a Christian, and it didn't take long in our dialogue to get confirmation. They wouldn't linger too long, respecting my desire to talk to the "other side"—the agnostics and even atheists brave enough to converse with me. Sometimes these believers would ask for prayer or would pray for me. How nice.

The next type was the goofy curious. These were mainly teenagers or those in their early 20s who just wanted to have some fun, like stumping the professor with questions he could not possibly answer, such as "How old do you think I am?" or "What is my weight?" or really dumb questions like "What is my boyfriend's name?" They were delighted when I, of course, couldn't answer correctly, although

I would always try to have some fun with them by giving bizarre and funny answers. They thought it was a contest, testing the professor's knowledge, and they always won. But my goal was to start a dialogue. It didn't matter that I couldn't answer their questions.

The third type was comprised of the anti-religious ones. Their desire was to destroy any of my arguments and answers, though I never argued, along with trying to humiliate me and any semblance of religion. I loved dialoguing with them, no matter how angry or insulting they became. Sometimes I would be yelled at. Great. Let's draw a nice listening crowd. I loved telling them I was not religious at all, even though a person of faith, and that they were different: religion is man's invention; faith is from God. That stumped them. I'm not sure I reached any, but you never know.

Lastly, there were the genuinely curious and willing. These were what we might call the agnostics, or those who hadn't really thought about it. I had wonderful conversations with these folks and was often surprised by how many young people—even teenagers—fit into this open-minded category. Sometimes they would let me pray with or for them when I asked if I could. These might have been people who would drive by another day when I was foolishly out there and yell, "HEY PROFESSOR!" I loved it.

> **CAN WE TALK?**
>
> *Grace Math and Proving God.* In my search for means of integration of my science and psychology training and career with faith and God, I came across a book by M. Scott Peck, M.D., who wrote in his book *The Road Less Traveled* a chapter on grace. It is often defined as the unmerited or unearned favor of God. In other words, it means good things happen to you that you didn't earn and don't deserve. It's as Dave Ramsey says, "better than we deserve." Indeed. But rather than an amorphous spiritual truth, Peck defined it mathematically as well. He invoked probability theory, which states the law of averages will make just about all things even out in the end. Like a coin flip. Tails 50 percent, heads 50 percent.

> But how about bad things and good things happening to you? We live in a culture and are neurologically programmed to pay far more attention to the bad things that could harm us than the good things. So we count and track the bad things that happen, in part thanks to our wonderful "if it bleeds, it leads" media, and neglect many of the good things. So, a ratio, given that attention, would be at best half and half—half the times bad things will happen. But let's say we add to that proportion of good things, the bad things that *fail* to happen—the "near misses" so to speak. So, count all the good things that happen to you, add to them the bad things that *could* have and perhaps should have but didn't (a good thing), and compare that total to the bad things that actually *did* happen. What is your ratio of good to bad things, then? Is it 50/50? Think about it. It's not. It's probably more like a thousand good to one bad. Maybe a 60/40 or 70/30 ratio—defying logic. How can that be? It would violate the law of averages and probabilities! One viable explanation is the grace of God. There is a protective (maybe angelic?) force that keeps many bad things from happening that should and would otherwise happen, at least consistent with the law of probability and averages.
>
> *Suggestion:* Think about this when you are contemplating the possibility of God from a science perspective. I like to use this scientific probability grace explanation (along with the theoretical and scientific impossibility of evolution—that's for another book) in discussions with people to "prove" the existence and supernatural grace of God. My next book, on my radical, miraculous, supernatural experience with God, will address that more personally and in some detail. Keep an eye out for it, won't you?

Importantly, I would never do what too many other Christian evangelists would do, such as passing out tracts on the laws of salvation or imposing testimony on people who didn't ask for it. I haven't done ATP in a while, but probably will again. Hopefully soon.

Love Language

You've no doubt heard of the love languages or you should have. Dr. Gary Chapman and colleagues have written a celebrated book of the same title and have a companion program that goes along with it. You might check it out. If you search the internet, you'll find lots on it. But it has only been relatively recent that we in psychology were "permitted" to refer to something so amorphous and uncountable as "love"—much less to write about it. That was the pastor's deal, not ours.

Yet, when spirituality came more into the mainstream of psychological study, assessment, and therapeutic effectiveness, such as in the addictions, mindfulness meditation, and motivational counseling fields, it became acceptable for us psych types to delve into its study and application. Now we can talk about the spirit and spirituality, and even love, but that doesn't mean we have to or want to talk about God or religion—even though there has been a considerable amount written about the psychology of religion, all the way from St. Augustine through William James, Carl Rogers (a seminary-trained minister), and the popular professor, Jordan Peterson.

I'll let you check out the love languages on your own. Let it just be said that we all have them, our own preferences and means of expressing and receiving love. Remember I discussed that the Type A intervention that worked with the angry, highly stressed, and joyless ("spiritually bankrupt") strivers seemed to be helping them learn to give and receive love. Amazing.

CAN WE TALK?

The OTHER Love Languages. You've probably all heard about the love languages—you know, acts of service, loving gifts, physical touch, words of encouragement, and so on. All good stuff for love, relationships, and especially marriage. But what about those "languages" *not* written about or as well-known and appreciated. Might I try?

Spiritual Integration Crossroads

Here are a few others for those of us who need some extra help with loving. They are my creations, so don't blame Dr. Chapman and colleagues—they had nothing to do with the following and no doubt *want* nothing to do with them! They are hereby released of all connection or liability.

Face Time. This is not the Apple iPhone thing, though it could apply to that as well. It has to do with the critical nature of your facial expressions. You've probably heard that quasi-idiotic estimate that 80 or 90 percent of all communication and interaction is nonverbal. I never could find out who came up with that figure and what so-called research it was based on. Probably little or none. But those nonverbals do play a pretty important role in how our communication is received and processed *by others*—even 20 percent would be significant. Nevertheless, let's agree that a lot of what we communicate to another does not have to do with our words. It's our facial expression.

Here's an experiment: Try holding your head still, looking straight at the person when you are talking—no nodding or moving. It's hard and maybe impossible for you. Conversely, there are the folks who shake their head no as they are verbally agreeing or saying yes to something. The police call this a "tell." It can mean the opposite of what they are saying, i.e., a lie or untruth. Look for it in yourself and others. It happens. If you've committed a crime, or are thinking about such, hold your head steady when being interviewed or interrogated by a spouse or the FBI. Both can detect your tells, so be very careful!

Suggestion: Clearly, our nonverbal expression is important. Depending on your goal, it may get you in trouble and communicate the opposite of what you are trying to say. Here are some suggestions for you.

Smile. No matter what you are saying—unless you are purposely wanting to communicate that you are angry or upset—smile. Those facial muscles involved in smiling (the zygomatic ones) make you feel better as well. I once had a colleague who would punctuate each of his statements with a smile at the end. We knew he was done with that thought. My other colleague and I noticed and liked it. It's a love language "trick" that can go a long way toward promoting positive communication and love. By the way, the evil lip purse or smirk fits into the category of non-smile. A smile cures these.

Suggestion: Smile to begin each of your communications, and smile as a period at the end of your statements. Do this especially when expecting or engaged in a disagreement.

Eye Roll Prevention. Did you know that what we don't do can have an even more critical effect on our loving communications? It's true, and Professor John Gottman would agree about this one—the contemptuous eye roll (along with the lip purse). It's tough to suppress this unloving behavior, especially if you are in the habit, but it's not impossible. Here are some ideas for you.

Suggestion: Try these: fake a sneeze (closing your eyes, of course), or look down as if looking for something on the floor, lower your head, or bury it in your hand or tissue. Or immediately upon detecting the beginning of an eye roll response, open your eyes wide and look past or to the left or right of the offending partner, as if you saw something crazy, fascinating, or scary. When questioned, say you thought you saw something over there. Helpful? I know, brilliant ideas. You are welcome. (By the way, I'm hoping my wife or your significant other does not read this section. Once they know what you are doing, they won't work.)

Criticism Blocking. This common communication toxicity is also a very hard one to stop. We all do it. Criticism is the number one Horseman of the Apocalypse that if unharnessed can undermine your love language, positive communication, and even your relationship as a whole. Sure, you could put duct tape over your mouth, and that would work, but looks weird. But how about stopping in the middle, apologizing, and taking back the criticism, or putting yourself in timeout away from the person you are wanting to or are actually criticizing until

> the urge or anger passes. Look in the mirror. I'm guessing you do lots of things that could be criticized. There also is the do-over in which you ask to say over and fix what you said wrongly. Then there is the start-over, where you literally leave the room, come back in, and (with a nice smile) say the opposite, positive thing. *Acting as if* is another way to stop or avoid criticizing, but if all this does not work, the issues are much deeper, and the anger and unforgiveness greater. That's when therapy can help.
>
> *Prayer.* Finally, if you are a person of faith and believe in prayer (or even if you are not!), try prayer before and possibly during your communication with the offending suspect. I sometimes encourage clients to pray before coming together and talking, especially over difficult subjects. There also is something I learned from a therapist couple called "rolling" or "conversational" prayer. For example, in the middle of a discussion where you are messing up or not sure what to say, roll right into prayer such as: "God, I am really struggling to communicate with X right now and we are both kind of upset. Please help us to understand each other, to be better at listening and not reacting so much," and so on. It can really work.
>
> Good luck with these "other" love languages. I believe Chapman and his colleagues will forgive me for adding these to the love language conversation. Practice them until they become more automatic. It's possible and they work!

Clinical Practice Integration

My focus on integrating my faith and psychology extended naturally to my clinical practice as I've been describing, but there were several areas that my counseling focused on and drew from, including addiction (Gerald May in his book *Addiction and Grace* states that all dependencies on anything but God are addictions), and W. R. Miller[23] has written powerfully on agape love as a key component of the motivational and healing process of therapy. Importantly, forgiveness (especially biblically driven), motivation, and change all have critical spiritual components that are strongly evidence and clinical validation supported. Each has essential spiritual aspects worthy of powerful attention.

Forgiveness
In my work with couples mainly, the topic of forgiveness usually comes up and needs to be addressed for relationship healing, if not saving. Forgiveness is an active process that usually doesn't happen on its own, or happens passively over time, and both the secular therapeutic science and the Bible offer rationales and strategies for dealing with the harm of unforgiveness and bitterness. You have probably heard the phrase, "Time heals all wounds," and unforgiveness indeed causes heart and relationship wounds. In fact, the evidence is clear that "time" heals *no* wounds.

I remember a time when I was speaking in a 12-Step meeting about something that I had done and that I felt guilt and shame about when a dear friend named Dottie (an ex–drug addict whose life was totally transformed by God through the 12-Step program) confronted me! Now those of you who know about the appropriate behavior in those meetings appreciate that *no one* interrupts when a person is sharing their "experience, strength, and hope." But Dottie didn't care. Her powerful love and empathy elbowed its way past decorum and she yelled at me: "DID YOU CONFESS THIS TO GOD?" My answer: yes. "HAS HE FORGIVEN YOU FOR WHAT YOU HAVE DONE?" (The whole large meeting now turning their heads back and forth between Dottie and me, as if watching a tennis match.) Yes. "THEN WHO ARE **YOU** NOT TO FORGIVE YOURSELF. **ARE YOU GOD?**" Wow. It was as if I'd been hit with a sledgehammer in my chest. I never forgot that emotional tennis match with Dottie. Learn to love and forgive yourself, especially through loving and forgiving others, and, of course, receiving and believing in God's love and forgiveness.

We know that forgiveness—a letting go of bitterness, resentment, and even blame—has important physical health benefits as well. People who forgive, or are more likely to forgive offenses, live longer, happier (duh), and healthier lives. Period. The opposite is true: those who don't are more likely to get sick and die younger.

I envisioned forgiveness as a three-stage *process*, including, (A) decision to forgive, (B) confession of unforgiveness, bitterness, and blame, and (C) the forgiving steps. Unfortunately, many seem to only employ the first step or stage and not the second or third. The church can be equally negligent of the full process as those in the secular world.

The first stage is the decision to forgive, to *decide* to let go of the offense and bitterness, resentment, and blame. Deciding and committing to forgive is the necessary start—but then the stepwise process is required to complete the healing. The steps I would help lead couples through—hopefully prayerfully with believers and faith-based relationships, but not necessarily—included:

1. **Exposing**, declaring, exposing, and owning what happened—what was done against you that you have been holding offense and blame over. This can take time and should not be hurried, but the person or couple should not set up permanent "camp" there—as many unfortunately do.

2. **Confessing** what *you* did with it (as harmful to yourself and the other). Unforgiveness has been described as drinking poison (of bitterness) and hoping the other person will die. The Bible states that forgiveness is more for the benefit of the unforgiving one than the one who caused the harm, but it is for both as well.

3. **Forgiving.** There are three important parts to this forgiving component—declaring (specifically, in front of God and another) forgiveness of the other and for what exactly you are forgiving them of. This includes the commitment to no longer hold them to blame or responsible for the hurt or harm to the forgiver. I note the Lord's prayer: "Forgive me *as* I forgive others…"

Secondly, asking God to forgive you for holding unforgiveness and bitterness against the other person. This could include asking one's partner, face-to-face, for their forgiveness for becoming bitter and unforgiving.

Thirdly, deciding to forgive yourself and no longer holding things against yourself. Guilt and shame can and should be released here at this step. Sometimes (no, *oftentimes*) people are too harsh with themselves, believing the words spoken or things done against them and becoming their own worst enemy. I encourage clients (and myself) to focus on and practice the latter part of the Great Commandment Jesus gave us: "…love others *as you love yourself*." And it's not possible to love others very well (or at all) if you do not love, or if you hate, yourself. Forgiving oneself, especially by going through these forgiveness steps, may be an essential part of reaching that part of the commandment.

Interestingly (at least to me), a practice I've been following at least yearly is fasting and prayer. For up to seven days I will go away, for example, to a mountain cabin and not eat anything and only drink lemon water and a cup of coffee (I know you 40-day fasters, my 7-day fast is nothing compared to your 40-dayer, so pipe down and let me make my point). I find there is a huge amount of emotional and psychological (as well as physical) toxins that are released during this time alone, and I wonder if some of that is anger, self-blame, and unforgiveness toward myself.

Forgiveness does not mean an abusive or harmful person should be absolved of responsibility, or that the aggrieved person should continue to be around someone who continues to harm. In marriage, this can often be complicated, and there are myriad ways to address it.

4. **Healing.** This is the place where healing can now begin, including God's blessing and healing of the heart and relationships that have been wounded. People often are filled with guilt and shame over what they have done, or was done to them (including neglect), that they become closed off to any desire or ability to be healed. They don't "deserve" healing—to have a whole heart once again. At this step, after getting honest with self and God and another, confessing wrong (James 5:16 in the Bible captures this), and giving and receiving forgiveness (the Lord's prayer as well), heart and life healing can then begin. The resistance wall crumbles or melts. Sometimes it takes forgiving oneself to get to the true healing step. The Christian faith teaches that *no* one deserves to be forgiven or healed by God (or others?)—but that is where unearned grace enters and works.

Finally, the effective result of the three forgiveness exercises enables healing in the person. Recall that in the successful RCPP type

A treatment study, it was when the heart disease men learned and practiced loving self and others that the change (and healing) came.

5. **Reconciling/Restoring** (when desired and possible). This is where the relationship can be repaired and restored, if wanted or needed. This reconciliation would not include an example such as a sexual molester (an uncle or family friend) who continues to be a danger, who has been forgiven but is not trustworthy to keep from offending once again.

Many couples are not ready or willing to go through this second phase or get stuck making their list of offenses and harms that are in need of forgiveness work and resolutions. My experience in therapy with individuals and especially couples is that roughly half never are able or willing to complete this three-stage and multiple-step process of forgiveness. Such an unnecessary misfortune. If they only knew.

Decide to forgive, then work on forgiving. It's hard to do, and for some, seemingly impossible. But it's not. The way we work with these resistant ones has a lot to do with how well we can "walk" with them through the process, from motivation to change.

Motivational counseling, or motivational interviewing[3-5], comes out of our newer science of motivation and change and has strong spiritual components—another opportunity for a collaboration between and integration of faith and science. There is much writing on this, including mine[24-28], and I have provided a number of illustrations of my using these motivational approaches with my clients and ministries in this book so far. There are many training programs and trainers available for those in the psychology, ministry, and therapy fields, which now includes the criminal and rehabilitation areas of corrections, probations officers, and prison counselors. (See www.motivationalinterviewing.org.)

But the training for how to help those most resistant to changing is a complex, sophisticated, and potentially powerful process, and my article[24] on motivational interviewing and counseling adapted for the church and spiritual areas has addressed this only generally. I plan a much more detailed and expansive approach to this topic in a future book to be coming out soon.

> **CAN WE TALK?**
>
> *Correcting Motivationally without Correcting.* Correct someone without correcting and criticizing them? Yes. Here's how:
>
> You don't directly correct them, since this is usually felt by the corrected person as criticism, judgment, and pressure. And we know that doesn't work. What we do is come with a concern or something we notice and ask permission to share it. It might go something like this: "Would it be okay if I shared a concern I have about something I've noticed?" If you get a yes, then you can proceed, gently and carefully, while respecting their autonomy and freedom to receive what you are saying, or do something about it or not. It's a gentle correction, without directly correcting them. Try it and you'll find it can work, but it will take some practice, so don't be discouraged if at first you don't get the sort of response you want.
>
> *Suggestion: Collaborate, Don't Confront.* Your relationship with the person should be one of collaborative communication—a partnership, as it were—rather than a confrontation.

In general, we train people in motivational-style counseling and interviewing to avoid the following (which create resistance in people and pushes them away): (A) telling, directing, warning, judging, arguing, questioning, pressuring, and talking "at" the person from the pedestal of the "caring helper," "problem solver," or (God help them) "expert."

What is more positively motivational communication is: (B) asking, listening, accepting, focusing, evoking, reinforcing, and collaborating. Easy, right? Think again. This is hard. Which communication style is yours (A) or (B)? Don't answer that.

Our primary finding that motivation has a critical spiritual component of loving empathy summoned up from within the individual—not imposed programmatically upon him or her like many past programs—speaks to the church as well. Working motivationally with people is a collaborative process that is like gentle guidance, standing with them at a decision crossroads, and helping them decide what would be best for them, and then working with them on how to accomplish the desired changes—not preaching at them.

I recall a story I read or was told about a woman in church who demonstrated a powerful form of empathy and loving partnership or collaboration. She was a prayer partner who would pray for people after church at the altar, over their issues and hurts. The pastor noticed during one end of church time that his prayer partner and another lady were weeping together as they were praying, though, strangely, there didn't seem to be anything said especially by the prayer partner who was supposed to be praying. When they finished, the pastor asked his prayer partner what was so deeply troubling about the woman she was praying for. The prayer partner said, "I have *no* idea." She didn't need to know (and neither did the pastor) to realize a powerful healing encounter had occurred.

Another example of motivation coming out of deep empathy is from the Bible. When Job was covered with painful sores and boils, in which he even used a stone to scrape his skin off, his three friends displayed such a powerful form of empathy when they could only stand by, without saying a word for seven days (can you imagine), weeping for their friend Job. Now we know that after that, at least two of the three shifted to the judgment mode, and not surprisingly Job reacted negatively to their pleading declarations against him. Recall motivation science here on how and how not to motivate a person. Sometimes we get so close and then blow it.

> **CAN WE TALK?**
>
> *Empathy—The Loving Counseling and Communication Effect: What Is It and How Do You Get It?* Empathy is neither a gift nor a given. It is a characteristic of positive communication and typically has to be learned. Empathy is an expression of the heart, of love and care, not so much just a feeling state, that effects and affects others

> in powerful ways. It is considered the core of what makes motivational counseling and interviewing work so well in helping people feel accepted and motivated toward positive change (not judged or pressured), and it requires skillful expressive behaviors. Some people are good at it, and others are not, and it's not just a matter of *feeling* caring toward another—it must be *expressed!* Empathy includes what not to do and say, for example telling, directing, analyzing too much, questioning, warning, and arguing for change are all non-empathic forms of blocking positive communication.
>
> *Suggestion:* Spend time learning how to be more empathic with others. Get training in reflective listening and communicating. Stop doing so much of those things that restrict or block empathy, like constantly telling and directing people, pressuring them, arguing or questioning them, or judging their behavior and motives. Come alongside them to listen (the Bible says to be quick to listen and slow to speak—learn to do that. It takes much practice!) rather than pushing them from behind or pulling on them from ahead. It's one of the best ways to express love and care, motivationally.

To feel the love of a person through their expressed empathy and God at the same time is an amazingly uplifting and positive motivational experience. In my work with individuals and couples, as well as mission work in the church, I've applied this motivational style to communication and approaches to changing that are spiritually related and guided.

SEVENTH FLOOR

PSYCHOLOGICAL REFLECTIONS

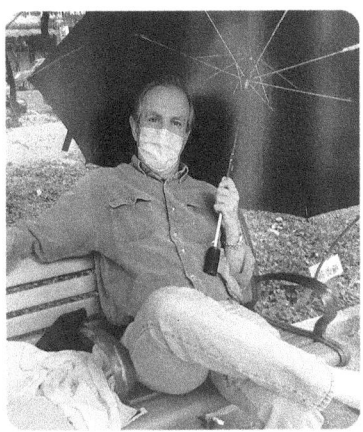

"There are far better things ahead than any we leave behind."

—C. S. Lewis

This final floor concludes the tour with a series of reflections to create a sort of closure to the reader with a final sense of life in and through psychology.

These last two chapters help us point to the "what now," "what's next," "whys and wherefores," and then final exit strategies and suggestions by your author-professor- guide.

Lastly, an author's postscript section is offered to those curiously and amazingly *still* interested in the how and why of the story of my writing of the book.

And, by the way, stopping with Room 800, or the Author Postscript—don't forget to go through the tour gift shop on the way out—your starving psychologists, therapists, and your author, of course, thank you.

ROOM 701

SO WHAT NOW?

"Is this the party with whom I am speaking?"
—Lily Tomlin (as Ernestine, the operator)

This book has been written for those interested in psychology, those already invested at some level in the field and practice, or those completely uninterested but, like my brother, daringly willing to attempt reading a funny, page-turning book about craziness in a field they shake their heads at and like making fun of—while at the same time (hopefully) learning a bit about psychology and the author they may not have wanted or needed to know—but now do.

Even after reading about my flights with insanity, trauma, PTSD, depression, anxiety, alcoholism, anger, and the rest, you may have wondered why I titled the book about a "crazy" professor and psychologist. Perhaps I should have been more circumspect or guarded about such an outright declaration—followed by all those evidences! It was not an exaggeration or device concocted to grab or hook you and others into buying (and hopefully reading) the book. It was actually an honest appraisal and descriptor of me and the book's stories. My use of self-deprecating humor was my guide to not make the book so heavy and dark. On the contrary, it is a hopeful book, filled with encouragement and light.

I was crazy, had gone crazy, and dealt with mental illness not just in others as a part of my field, but in a deeply personal way. I chose to tell the truth about my fight with insanity in as transparent and unvarnished a way as I could, and I hope you came to appreciate that I also wanted to give hope to others, since it is a hope-filled story, I believe, that healing and sanity is possible, no matter the difficulty of the path or barriers to health and life. I purposely intended this book to be one filled with humor, often the self-deprecating kind, and some "bathwater" truths about my field of psychology.

While not a religious book, I wanted to share my profound experience with God, such as what happens to an atheist professor who worshipped only at the altar of science and psychology when his life unravels and he has nowhere else to turn or fall—and the struggle to put the old life and career together with the new one. Do I stay in psychology or leave and follow God? If I stay, how in the world do I do that? What would it look like? Well, now you and I see. I trust you were not disappointed and got as much out of it all as I have in writing it. Some things can only be shared after you are retired from the former things (like professoring), as I am, are insulated from it, and it is not allowed to come back and bite you. I think I'm there. We shall see.

But I'm curious as to who has read this far. You have, haven't you? Are you a person already in the field, perhaps who knows me, wondering what revelations I made that included you? I've tried to be kind for the most part, and if I've got it wrong about you or us, please accept my apologies. It was not intended. Sometimes my hyperbole and sick sense of humor may have kicked you (but hopefully not), your field of psychology and practice, or shined a negative light on all that. Blame Dave Barry for my copied style of making fun of as much as possible, including you and me. I especially loved, as you have found, the use of ALL CAPS—something that worked far better for Dave than me!

Maybe you are someone considering a career in psychology. In the past, I've had numerous young or not-so-young people approach me with questions about how they could become a psychologist, therapist, or professor (just like me). The latter, who wanted my job, I would firmly rebuke with the statement and a smile—over my dead body will you get my job as a glorious, *tenured* (here I go again) professor. But no more for me, and those positions have long been filled by younger, no doubt much more competent, and less crazy folks. Go learn from them.

Remember the motivation science caution about giving anyone unsolicited advice and expecting them to receive, much less follow it?

So What Now?

I think it was Confucius who said, "Advice—wise people don't need it; fools won't heed it." I said that in the book, though you probably skipped or only skimmed that section. Here's some of my unsolicited advice to those of you semi-interested in the field of psychology or a career in it. Like lawyers, we already have a plethora of psychologists and therapists—a number of whom are unemployed, underemployed, or just not happy. Consider the field carefully, what division or type of psychology you want, and what you are "called" to pursue. Are you gifted and heart-felt directed to help others with their psychological, relationship, mental, and behavioral needs and problems? If not, run the other way! We don't need you, but might very much like to have you! (Not that I can speak for the field of psychology; please forgive me for giving you this unsolicited, kick in the rear advice. You did ask, didn't you?)

If you can't determine it, perhaps consider finding and pursuing another profession like welding or plumbing, maybe business school if you like, to make money (just not advertising!). These skills can be excellent, highly rewarding both financially and personally, and with full employment opportunities everywhere in the world. Regarding advertising, I'm kidding (mostly)—I'm still struggling with bad karma from my dad's "evilness" as a mad man selling useless stuff and sometimes even disease to and on us. Keep me posted on what you decide.

If you are a student, *why?* Figure that out first, why you need to be there. If you can't come up with a good reason, then find one, or spend some time seeking out what you are good at, what you love doing, and pursue it. There are professional and not-so-professional coaches and "encouragers" all over that will offer help. I used a terrific one who happened to be a friend whom I met on the Romania mission trip, Dave Thorpe, who does professional coaching to any who are stuck in life or who want more out of it. He has a website (www.path4success.com) and Facebook presence. Check him out. He helped me tremendously in my life directions and changes.

Remember my honest (drunk) student who dropped out of school and found the best job and career ever, that he wouldn't have found (ever, I believe) if he had been an excellent student and graduated with honors and all? Oh, all right, I'm not saying you shouldn't strive to be an excellent student and finish school, but you know what I mean (don't you?). While you might need to go to school to be able to do it, get a real paying job first, then invest in school if you need it and haven't lost your interest or desire by then. By the way, my son never finished college (I think he's three courses short) and never got his degree but went off and trained as a sports and body rehab specialist and is making more money than I made as a full professor! (It's not good to embarrass, okay, humiliate, your dad like that. Will someone who knows him please tell him that? Thank you.)

Continuing in *my* attempts to embarrass my dear family, case in point, my brother. After a number of ill-fated attempts at things school-like, he became a long- and short-haul trucker, car and cycle mechanic, and other life necessity work he won't admit to, he finally decided he wanted to work in the airplane industry. Any "sensible" person, not to mention egg-head professor like me, would have said: "Go back to school and figure out *there* what you want to do in life and *at least get your degree*! And good luck, by the way." But he already decided what he wanted to do! Wouldn't you know he boldly and stupidly marched into the aircraft company he had targeted for his future job and offered to do anything, at even the lowest pay, and was started figuratively sweeping the floors of the big factory. (I may be embellishing a bit here, but it is basically true.) He worked hard, learned the jobs just above each new pay grade and function, made himself too valuable an employee to be fired or let go, and finally after years and no formal education, was promoted to a white-collar engineering supervisor, over the quality control and jet engine mechanic training departments. Wow.

He's now in charge of training for all the engineers in this big company—a huge job with great responsibilities (imagine a poorly trained jet engine mechanic who, through shoddy work, causes a terrible plane crash. You got the idea). He didn't need to go back to school and certainly not waste his time wandering (and wondering, come to think of it) the "hallowed halls" of college or the university, being vomited out with no real job skills whatsoever—like so many of my students over the years.

Finally, if you are a person like my fun-loving, well-employed, hardworking brother David or son Josh, then continue to enjoy life at its fullest, drive your muscle and sports cars fast (and safely), but don't forget about what happens when you die. God knows and is there to help. Just ask.

Purpose

For all: live a life of purpose and meaning. If you don't have it, go find it, or at least invite it and open yourself up to it when it arrives. Or find someone like Dave Thorpe who can help you. Remember chaos theory: rigidity is disease, and healing comes from breaking it up first, then remaking. Consider God. He does a pretty good job with that. Consider me: flawed, broken, formerly rigid, transformed, happy. But how did I get from insane, psychology chaotic remaking to author and race-car driver (actually some truth in that; maybe another book—or obituary)?

Read on, if you like (or not), of my final parting (actually, imparting) thoughts to you, including meanderings on how and why I found my "writer man" within. Otherwise, it was fun talking with you and taking you on my tour of psychology. I hope we meet again.

> **FINAL TOUR/READER ALERT #3:** Be advised, our tour will come to an end as you are led through the psychology gift shop (did you think you were going to get away with skipping this standard tour money-grab?). Nevertheless, you are encouraged to please buy lots of things as you venture through it—weird psychological memorabilia, knickknacks, curios, and all—to help support your local starving psychologists, therapists, and teachers (my apologies to those psychologists and therapists who are *actually* starving for this *final* (thank God!) nasty attempt at humor).

ROOM 702

EXIT RIGHT— SOME FINAL PARTING THOUGHTS

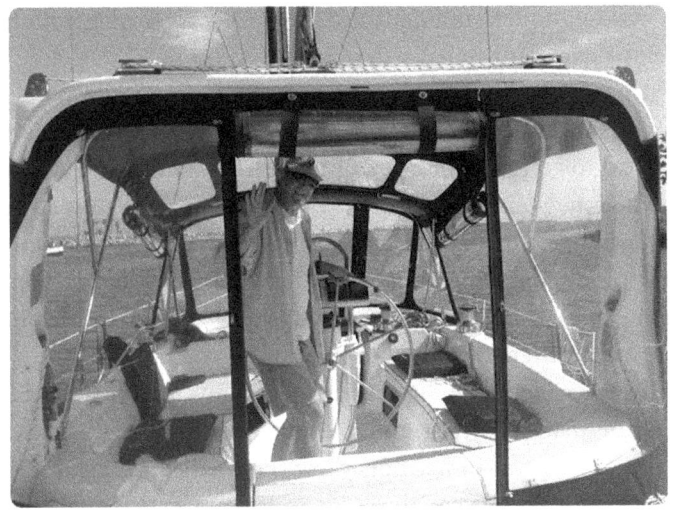

"Ahoy and Welcome Aboard!"
Ocean bound, starboard tack rights-of-way, glorious voyage ahead we lay.

"Life is a direction, not a destination."
—Carl Rogers

In my darkest days of marriage loss, depression, and addiction, I once had a dear friend, an older wiser woman in the AA program, confront me with love and understanding. I keenly remember the day when she curiously (to me) explained the difference between happiness and joy—neither of which I could possibly have been experiencing.

She had drawn my attention for some time with her grace and wisdom. I decided, I think, to make her my wise grandmother, though I never told her that and she may not have appreciated the elderness with which I had "blessed" her. I guess my heart, my new growing spirituality, and faith-to-be somehow recognized her presence as something special. I know now what it was but didn't then. I just knew, without understanding, I needed to have a meeting with her. It was a heart and spirit thing, a strange pull on both.

Then a powerful connection happened—ironically at a time when I was most depressed and broken down. During the meeting, I knew I had to go talk with her, so I made my way to her. I awkwardly approached and fumbled out my grave concern (I was usually good with words, but not that day) about my feelings of what I thought were happiness, bubbling up from my insides with clearly no apparent reasoning (I was quite unhappy in my life at the time). I was confused and not a little frightened by the sensation.

But she listened carefully and lovingly to my attempt at explaining my fear of that unknown and irrational feeling. Then she smiled with love at me, and in her honeydew Southern drawl educated me: "Honey, why that's not happiness, that's JOY." My response: "But I've done nothing to be happy about. My life is a mess, and I could *not* be happy. Why does it feel like that?" Her retort: "Joy is a gift from God. You can't earn it or deserve it. He just gives it to you because He loves you."

I never forgot that discussion. Actually, it was more of a loving impartation. I've shared it with many, and now y'all too. It was like I was speaking with God's special angel, placed there for me, and that moment. Has something like that ever happened to you? I'm guessing for many of you readers, it has.

But I have one last section for those of you who are interested enough in how your author got from retired professor to (creative) writer—that implausible transition that led me down a final (I think, but who knows?) newer crooked path to professing before unforced non-students like you.

ROOM 800
(OPTIONAL BONUS—OR PUNISHMENT)

AUTHOR POSTSCRIPT: FROM ACADEMIC TO WRITER

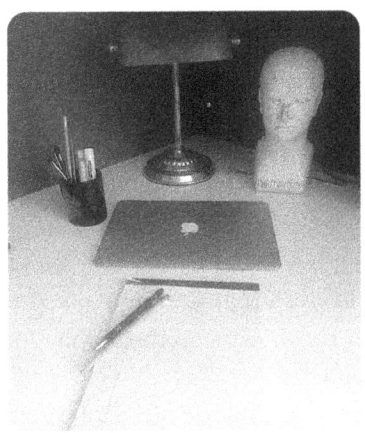

"Nobody ever committed suicide while reading a good book, but many have while trying to write one."

—Robert Byrne

Discovering My *What* and *Why Now*

This final postscript psychology confidential section is offered for those wondering about my path from professor and psychologist to creative writer—how and why (especially) I got from there to here.

My rigid life as a teacher and professor, nearing rigor mortis according to my friends, was broken up in a familiar chaotic mess of "healing variability" as I was ushered to the academic door I once had dragged myself through. I can't say I was so successful avoiding the door hitting me on the way out. It did. Then it was a "now what?" And writing was not my first or even second option.

It wasn't the first time I tried divorcing psychology, like I had with my marriages. Psychology just wouldn't let me go. But now it had, with my reluctant cooperation and a cliff-hanging (mother eagle–like) shove from God. Somehow, through a strange fusion of both bad and good fortune, with a bolus of opportunistic providence, I made it all the way through that psychological wormhole to full, tenured professor. It was the pinnacle! Or so I thought. Then, it was in the rearview mirror.

Private psychological practice happened and brought a hopeful blending of the spiritual and the clinical, while paying for those persistent bills. But the hand of God pulled me further away, though never entirely, from life in psychology. It was a little like the time I first set foot on the tarmac at the airport in Johannesburg, South Africa, when an unfamiliar passion (some say a "calling") overcame me, followed by my nine trips there for teaching, doing community health research, serving, loving, and being loved by the people of Africa. But life and love of writing? Yeah, right.

Nevertheless, writing commenced painfully for one so unscripted in this new discipline. Here was the vision that wouldn't leave me alone: "Surviving Psychology" (the previous title) and finally *Psychology Confidential* was to be a story of my wild and crazy path to and through the world of psychology, what happened, and how I and those closest to and affected most by me more or less survived.

I had a good deal of fun, lots of adventure, as well as needed encounters of humbling—and often necessary humiliating—experiences and confessions. I wanted also to help the reader consider lowering that psychological pedestal you put us up on—or in contrast, lift us up from that pit you threw us down into after we "abused" you with bad grades, brain-frazzling confusions, gross unhelpfulness, philosophical and psychological babble, or just extreme boredom. We psych purveyors became good at it all—since we *had* to be in order to survive the ordeal ourselves—and then, of course, to pass it on to you.

Looking back as this twice-retired psychology professor, teacher, mentor, and researcher, still "young" in my early 60s when I began my quest to write about it, I found myself thinking for a good while about what in the world to do next. I was pretty sure I was done with the *professorial* life—a conclusion a number of others had reached on my behalf (friends and foes alike)—but now what? One thought that nagged at me, like a dissatisfied, unfulfilled wife, was whether to share with the world my strange, crooked life path to and through psychology—traumas, insanity, and all. An editor I worked with once cautioned me about writing about myself. "Even God only had one book written about him" and a friend questioned whether I should write in the first person about myself. I was indeed ambivalent. Who would be interested in a story like mine (besides, of course, *me*)? And who could I recruit to write about wonderful me and my amazing life story? You guessed it: no one.

Ambivalence and any semblance of humility shoved aside, like an uppity forward crowding the crease in front of the goalie I was protecting as a hockey defenseman, I decided to begin writing. What could it hurt? It certainly was an easy fit with my great self-centeredness.

Besides tracing my strange path to and through the world of psychology, I've woven throughout—you might say, "spiced it up"—with stories of my weird but funny family, our series of goofy dogs and cats, some pretty significant personal traumas, and a variety of experiences with some amazing people I've known and come across in my life and career. I included some of my world travels as a psychologist, professor/teacher, and researcher to East Germany, Africa, and Asia, among other places where my life in psychology took me.

When I finally exited academia (or rather was unceremoniously, though relatively happily, led out the same door I had weirdly entered 40 years previously), one wise friend told me: "Well, it's about time. We've known for a good while you needed to get out of there!" Indeed. I was burned out, discouraged, and needed a change. My relationships and living spaces were stuck in that same place as well. It was like God was shaking things up that needed to be broken up, starting with yanking that academe pedestal I had propped myself upon out from under me.

But there I was with too much time on my hands, retired, more or less, and I confess, with bills still to pay. At least I could grow my private practice as a licensed clinical psychologist. I kept my license current, maybe as a "fall back," but never much used it. But now I needed it. That should have been enough: apply my skills and experience to other lives and relationships, even or especially the kinds I never was so good at myself. And so I did, for better or worse.

Nonetheless, the idea of writing wouldn't leave me be, and I came to that notion, perhaps I could write about some of those crazy stories and experiences I had in and through a long career in psychology. My overgrown, self-centered ego pictured sort of an Insider Tells All! (see subtitle)—the "Evil Underbelly of Psychology"—as told by me. You bet.

But this was not the kind of writing I was used to. I could and did write research articles, teaching presentations, psychological research findings, study methods and such, to students, the public, or colleagues. This other kind of writing was different, more like creative writing, blending professional experiences with personal stories.

There were all those strange, often funny experiences I found myself sharing with buddies during long bike rides, marathon training runs, sailing voyages, or just having coffee or a beer together. Probably most significantly, about 10 years ago I had this precious female friend and then fiancée—now passed on after a heroic but losing battle with cancer—who seemed so touched, tickled, delighted, or shocked by a variety of these my-life-in-and-out-of-psychology with crazy, personal, family, and animal stories—she would tell me I should put them in a book to share with others. Well, here it is, Lucia. Thank you, dear one. I'll see you again one day in heaven.

Thus, I began making notes on these various, sometimes bizarre, stories and experiences in and out of psychology. I especially added the stranger and more ridiculous ones from the personal arena that seemed to relate, not to mention adding to possible reader interest (and fabulous book popularity!). But how to write this sort of thing? It was a different animal for me to contemplate, much less tame and direct.

Then there were those two weird prayers and pray-ers (persons who prayed), I should say. Still struggling with my painful and unceremonious release from the Professorial Dance Party, I found myself in recovery of sorts, seeking personal, relationship, and spiritual healing. I was visiting a church in Northern California—the charismatic kind where you could never tell what was going to happen next. They had lots of wild young people who seemed to believe *everything* in the Bible (strange, huh?) and that they were free to speak words from God into perfect strangers. Me.

On two completely separate occasions and days, two different young persons asked to pray for me, and both independently told me I was a *writer*. Yes, I told them, I had written a number of things, research articles, grants, book chapters. That sort of stuff. But that was not what they meant. They even used the term *creative* for the kind of writing I would do. I won't tell you what else they said. We shall see if that comes true. I guess you readers will be the deciders ultimately.

But the writing itself was the bigger wall. Deciding was one thing. The next was the *how*. I knew how to apply behavioral psychology to a task like that and so I tried: place learning! You readers who have actually *read* the book will recall one of my Can We Talk? asides on stimulus control and creating a habit. Simple, right? Nope.

I created a great place for writing (see picture) in my nice office at home, complete with timer and comfy (maybe too comfy) chair and all. Didn't work. I kept avoiding the office entirely! Then I decided to pull out the "big guns"—the punishment contract! (Remember the doctoral dissertation contract?) I decided on my good friend Dave—just mean enough and a good enough friend—to implement and enforce the contract. I had to write so many hours (and words per week) or I would have to donate a significant amount of money to three most hated organizations. But Dave and his wife were not that keen on helping (or forcing would be a better word) me to write something that should be done because I wanted to, had a passion for. They were right. I didn't do the contract. By the way, I'm not going to tell you which most hated organizations I chose. But then what?

I'm thinking it was the grace of God and in answer to my prayers for help that I found Paper Raven Books (PRB) and Morgan Gist

MacDonald. She had written one of (if not *the*) best-selling books on how to write a book in a short period of time (thanks also to my friend and award-winning novelist and writing teacher, Randy Ingermanson, for his help), and I found out about their special needs program (lol) for helping would-be authors like me, to write and *finish* a book! Thanks to PRB, Morgan, and other great editors, including James and Brian, I made it. It was like a breakthrough in which I went from having to force myself to sit down and write, to wanting to write. I had a passion. And here we are, at the finish line.

My original title for the book, once I began *actually* writing and not just making random notes or drafts, was "PSYCH Matter." I decided I wanted to name it after one of my favorite personal biographies that gave an inside account of the personal, professional, and spiritual struggle of an eminent neurosurgeon. But in Dr. David Levy's book, *Gray Matter*, he described his life becoming and operating as a specialist neurosurgeon fearfully but effectively introducing prayer in his practice. You might have seen after reading this one why his book was such an inspiration to me and my writing here. "PSYCH Matter" then turned into "Psychologized," followed by "Surviving Psychology," and now *Psychology Confidential*. (You'd think I could make up my darn mind, but this captured it best, don't you think after reading it? You *did* read it, didn't you? or are you cheating and turning ahead to the last chapter to find out the end of the story? I sincerely hope not.)

My spiritual transformation from science- and psychology-worshipping professor to God-believing professor worshipping at a different altar attempted to tell a similar kind of story of a professional/spiritual integration as *Gray Matter* illustrated. *Psychology Confidential* was written to unlock and describe the inner and outer worlds of one who had traveled the gamut of nearly all the various roles a psychologist could ever play, and then who experienced (and survived) a radical religious conversion. Dr. Levy was the head surgeon; I was the headshrinker, crazy professor, and (called by colleagues and none other than my mother) "religious fundamentalist," and "Jesus freak!"

The stories and remembrances I ultimately decided to include traced my more or less crooked life and professional path, and the many intended and especially unintended consequences and blessings, through my radical fight integrating faith with profession and psychology along the way. I hope that its blender-mix of those personal, professional, spiritual, and relationship stories, breakdowns, and breakthroughs; animal fun; and world travels made for good reading and possibly occasional (or accidental) learning, if not sheer entertainment—all from your psychology "answer man's" perspective on the inner and outer workings of a life shot through the prism of a world of psychology, family, faith, and fun.

Warmly,

Dr. John

John E. Martin, Ph.D.
Spring 2021

How can we understand the road we travel? It is the LORD who directs our steps (and path).
—Proverbs 20:24

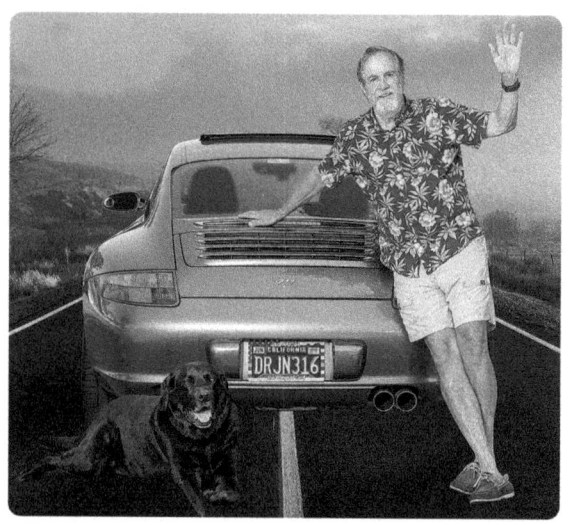

Dr. John and Barnabas (Velo), his wonderful Lab and service/companion canine wishing you
"So long and God speed"

on your own *Road Less Traveled* journey.

MORE ABOUT DR. JOHN

Dr. Martin's career has spanned 40+ years since he first began work as a master's-level child psychologist and special education teacher in 1972. Two master's degrees later, he earned his doctorate in Clinical Psychology in 1978. Since then, he has served on the faculties at universities, medical schools, and centers, including the Jackson VA and University of Mississippi Medical Center, Belhaven University and Millsaps College, San Diego State University and University of California, San Diego School of Medicine, Faccoschule Magdeburg (Germany), and Universities of Johannesburg, Rand Afrikaans, and Stellenbosch (South Africa), and finally as Professor of Clinical Psychology at Fuller Theological Seminary Graduate School of Psychology.

John has published over 70 articles in scientific journals, two books, and various book chapters, including over 100 professional presentations at scientific organizations in addictions, health psychology, and behavioral medicine, as well as motivational counseling application to the church ministries.

Supporting his work in clinical psychology and behavioral medicine research, he received more than $2 million in US and state of California grants, specifically in the areas of addictions, smoking, and health and disease risk modification. He is a Fellow in several psychology and behavioral medicine societies, having served as Associate Editor and on the editorial and review boards of numerous scientific journals, including National VA and NIH grant review sections.

A Christian since 1984, after experiencing a powerful transformative experience with God, John has additionally served in various church ministries, currently as an active member of a large nondenominational, evangelical Christian church in Southern California (cottonwood.org), where he graduated from their two-year School of Ministry/Leadership College.

For more detailed history of John's professional life, see www.johnmartinphd.com.
Readers interested in communicating with John, can email: drjohn@psychologyconfidentialthebook.com.

ACKNOWLEDGEMENTS

I am grateful to those special people who have influenced, guided, taught, stimulated, collaborated with and encouraged me in my professional and personal life, as well as for their feedback on this book about my life in psychology.

Several lived through it with me, such as Rebecca, mainly, but also Lucia and Catherine. Others were strong supporters and at times helpful editors, including Chris Cecil, longtime friend and fellow writer, Patti, Ken, and the Blue crew—my "second family" during a trying time—as well as my coffee and bike-riding buddies Steve Henning, Guy Gilchrist, Mike Koch, and Bob Rivera. Finally, there are my special friends and chief encouragers, Dave Thorpe, Gerry Lumba, and my amazing son, Josh Martin.

There were those powerful spiritual nudges—pushes, really—from God and His own at Bethel Church in Redding, CA, from whom I received those prophetic prayers that made such a big difference in my decision, conviction, and motivation to write, especially what I've shared herein. I thank God I said yes.

I thank my four primary mentors who guided me through different phases in my development as a psychologist, clinician, researcher, and teaching professor: David A. Sachs (master's), James Fitch (master's), Leonard H. Epstein (doctoral), and William R. Miller, (post-doc, and my close friend, colleague, spiritual integrator, and wise counselor). While they may not want this acknowledgement, I think they will forgive me for all the weird psychology and strange stories I've promulgated—for which they bear little or no personal responsibility or fault. Hopefully, they will get some enjoyment, or experience some positive recollections at least, in their telling. Nevertheless, I am most appreciative of their positive role in my professional development and life directions.

On the flip side, I have taught, mentored, and collaborated with many outstanding students, colleagues, and clinical interns (too many to mention here), and would like to acknowledge the following for their positive role in my career, life, and many successes I have had as a teacher, clinical supervisor, researcher, and professor of psychology: Pat Dubbert, Christi Patten, Don Prue, Bob Kaplan, Al Litrownik, Jim Sallis, Lee Frederiksen, Terry Keane, Jeff Webster, Karen Calfas, Heidi Squier Kraft, Scott Walters, Jim Noto, Mark Myers, Paul Cinciripini, Debbie Ossip-

Klein, Frank Collins, Ed Wolff, Kevin Thompson, John Fairbank, Neil Johnson, Alan Katell, Jim Fitterling, Abby King, Tim Ahles, Jenifer Booth, Alex Mijares, Shaun Wehle, John Lee, Priscilla Sihn, Mariam Baim, Stephanie Smolinski, and especially Ellie Sturgis, Randy Ingermanson, Don and Annie Walker, my business associate, Vip Patel, as well as those critical spiritual mentors, colleagues, pastors and friends—Charlie Carlson, Bill Miller, Ken Blue, Joe Ozawa, Kenneth Mulkey, Dan Kotoff and Siang-Yang Tan.

I am grateful to my beta reviewers who agreed (some foolishly), volunteered, or were involuntarily drafted to be initial reviewers of an unfinished draft of the book. These brave readers included friends, two conscripted ("fact check") family members, and willing professional associates. For their help in my effort to craft a decent book worth reading, I thank Catherine, Josh and David Martin, Ps Fred May, Mike Koch, Jode' Hyman, and John Watkins for their both useful and useless (lol) feedback, suggestions, *warnings* (!), and any hopeful encouragement—that is, that I can actually make it barely readable in the end. In a weak gesture of appreciation, each will have received the first hot-off-the-presses, exceptionally valuable, signed copies of the final hardcover to bury somewhere in their dusty bookshelves (for posterity reasons, of course).

Finally, I thank Paper Raven Books and my special editors including Morgan Gist MacDonald, James Ranson, and Brian Dooley, among the many others at PRB who helped tremendously to organize, form, and craft this book. Then there were my close friends, Don Lace and Jode' Hyman, who gave me the idea for the book title—*Psychology Confidential*. Thank you, Jo. It was your dinner imagination that dropped the perfect description and title on me—after months (years actually) of my searching for it.

I gratefully acknowledge and extend my deep thankfulness to each of you for your friendship, encouragement, caring, and often prayerful support, on my path to finally writing and finishing *Psychology Confidential*, my own life craziness, and ultimately learning (sort of) to be a different kind of writer and person.

REFERENCES

1 Martin, J. E. & Sachs, D. A. (1973). The effects of visual feedback on the fine motor behavior of a deaf cerebral palsied child. *Journal of Nervous and Mental Disease*, 157, 59-62

2 Martin, J. E., Epstein, L. H. & Cinciripini, P. M. (1980). Effects of feedback and stimulus control on pulse transit time discrimination, *Psychophysiology*, 17, 431-436.

3 Miller, W. R. & Rollnick, S. (1993). *Motivational Interviewing: Preparing People to change addictive behavior*. NY: Guilford Press.

4 Miller, W. R. & Rollnick, S. (2003). *Motivational Interviewing: Preparing people to change* (2nd Edition). NY: Guilford Press.

5 Miller, W. R. & Rollnick, S. (2013). *Motivational Interviewing*: 3rd Edition. Helping People Change. NY: Guilford Press.

6 Prue, D. M., Krapfl, J. E. & Martin, J. E. (1981). Brand fading: The effects of gradual changes to low tar and nicotine cigarettes on smoking, rate, carbon monoxide and thiocyanate levels. *Behavior Therapy*, 12, 400-416.

7 Martin, J. E., Calfas, K. J., Patten, C. A., Polarek, M., Hofstetter, R., Noto, J., & Beach, D. (1997). Prospective evaluation of three smoking interventions in 205 recovering alcoholics: One- year results of Project SCRAP-tobacco. *Jr. of Consulting and Clinical Psychology, 65,* 190-948

8 Patten, C. A., Martin, J. E., Hofstetter, R., Brown, S. A., Kim, N., & Williams, C. D. (1999). Smoking cessation following a smoke-free Navy alcohol rehabilitation program, *Journal of Substance Abuse Treatment,* 16, 61-69.

9 Patten, C. A., Martin, J. E., Calfas, K. J., Brown, S. A., & Schroeder, D. R. (2000). Effects of three smoking cessation treatments on nicotine withdrawal in 141 abstinent alcoholic smokers. *Addictive Behaviors, 25, 301-306.*

10 Patten, C. A., Martin, J. E., Myers, M. G., Calfas, K. J., & Williams, C. D. (1998). Effectiveness of cognitive-behavioral therapy for smokers with histories of alcohol dependence and depression. *Journal of Studies on Alcohol, 59,* 327-335.

11 Martin, J. E. (Chair). (1979). Marketing Health. Association for Advancement of Behavior Therapy, San Francisco.

12 Martin, J. E. & Frederiksen, L. W. (December 1979). Marketing behavioral medicine services in a hospital setting. Association for Advancement of Behavior Therapy, San Francisco.

13 Walters, S. T., Miller, E., & Chiauzzi, E. (2005). Wired for wellness: e-Interventions for addressing college drinking. *Journal of Substance Abuse Treatment,* 29:205 139-145.

14 Martin, J. E., Dubbert, P. M., Katell, A. D., Thompson, J. K., Raczynski, J. R., Lake, M., Smith, P. O., Webster, J. S., Sikora, T., & Cohen, R. E. (1984). The behavioral control of exercise in sedentary adults: Studies 1 through 6. *Journal of Consulting and Clinical Psychology, 52,* 795-811.

15 Martin, J. E., Dubbert, P. M., & Cushman, W. C. (1985). Controlled trial of aerobic exercise in hypertension. *Circulation,* 72: III-13, Supp III.

16 Dubbert, P. M., Martin, J. E., Zimering, R. T., Burkett, P. A., Lake, M., & Cushman, W. C. (1984). Behavioral control of mild hypertension with aerobic exercise: Two case studies. *Behavior Therapy,* 15, 373-380.

17 Martin, J. E., Wolff, E., Patten, C. A., Squier, H., Caparosa, S., Beach, D., Slymen, D., Bastos, E., Heys, S., & Lutschmann, R. (March 1996). Cross-Cultural evaluation of exercise effects on elder hypertensives. Presentation before Society of Behavioral Medicine and International Congress of Behavioral Medicine, Washington D.C.

18 Ahles, T. A., King, A. C., & Martin, J. E. (1984). EMG biofeedback during dynamic movement as a treatment for tension headache. *Headache,* 24, 41-44.

19 Fitterling, J. M., Martin, J. E., Gramling, S., Cole, P., & Milan, M. A. (1988). Behavioral management of exercise training in vascular headache patients: An investigation of exercise adherence and headache activity. *Journal of Applied Behavior Analysis,* 21, 9-19.

20 Martin, J. E. & Sachs, D. A. (1973). The effects of a self-control weight loss program on an obese woman. *Journal of Behavior Therapy and Experimental Psychiatry,* 4, 155-159.

21 Miller, W. R. & C'de Baca, J. (2002) Quantum change: When epiphanies and sudden insights transform ordinary lives, *Journal of Psychiatry and Law,* 30 (3): 395-399.

22 Martin, J. E., & Miller, W. R. (Co-Chair). (November 1984). Integrating Behavioral and Spiritual Approaches to Behavior Change. Association for advancement of Behavior Therapy, Philadelphia.

23 Miller, W. R. (2000). Rediscovering fire: Small interventions, large effects. *Psychology of Addictive Behaviors,* 14 (1), 6-18.

24 Martin, J. E. & Sihn, E. P. (2009). Motivational interviewing: Applications in Christian therapy and church ministry. *Journal of Psychology and Christianity.,* vol. 28, no. 1, pp. 71-77.

25 Miller, W. R., & Martin, J. E. (Eds.) (1988). *Behavior Therapy and Religion: Integrating Behavioral and Spiritual Approaches to Behavior Change:* Newbury Park, CA: Sage Press.

26 Booth, J., & Martin, J. E. (1998). Spiritual and religious factors in substance use, dependence and recovery. In H. Koenig (Ed.), *Handbook of Religion and Mental Health,* Academic Press: New York., 175-200

27 Martin, J. E., & Booth, J. (1999). Behavioral approaches to enhancing spirituality. In, W. R. Miller, *Spiritual and religious factors in counseling,* APA Publishing, Wash., D.C.

28 Martin, J. E., & Carlson, C. R. (1988). Spirituality and Health Psychology. In W. R. Miller, & J. E. Martin, *Behavior Therapy and Religion: Integrating Behavioral and Spiritual Approaches to Change,* Newbury Park, CA: Sage Press. 57-110.

General References

Arterburn, S., & Stoeker, F. (2020). *Every Man's Battle*. Colorado Springs: Waterbrook.

Kraft, H. S. (2007). *Rule Number Two. Lessons I Learned in a Combat Hospital.* New York: Little Brown.

Peck, M. Scott. (1983). *People of the Lie.* The Hope for Healing Human Evil. New York: Touchstone

Warren, R. (2002). *The Purpose Driven Life.* Grand Rapids, MI: Zondervan

www.ingramcontent.com/pod-product-compliance
Lightning Source LLC
Chambersburg PA
CBHW072224200426
43209CB00073B/1934/J